Biliary Tract - Review and Recent Progress

Edited by Qiang Yan and Zhiping Pan

Published in London, United Kingdom

Biliary Tract - Review and Recent Progress
http://dx.doi.org/10.5772/intechopen.102208
Edited by Qiang Yan and Zhiping Pan

Contributors
Diego Rossi Kleinübing, Sarah Luiz Brum, Laílson Alves Rodrigues, Umut Tüysüz, Mitzi Becerra, Magaly Torres, Beatriz Calderón, Iván Salinas, María Ruíz, Jorge Ventura, Alex Zendel, Yaniv Fenig, Alessandro Paniccia, Asmita Chopra, Qiang Yan, Zhiping Pan

First published in London, United Kingdom, 2023 by IntechOpen
IntechOpen is the global imprint of INTECHOPEN LIMITED, registered in England and Wales, registration number: 11086078, 5 Princes Gate Court, London, SW7 2QJ, United Kingdom

British Library Cataloguing-in-Publication Data
A catalogue record for this book is available from the British Library

Additional hard and PDF copies can be obtained from orders@intechopen.com

Biliary Tract - Review and Recent Progress
Edited by Qiang Yan and Zhiping Pan
p. cm.
Print ISBN 978-1-80356-698-6
Online ISBN 978-1-80356-699-3
eBook (PDF) ISBN 978-1-80356-700-6

Meet the editors

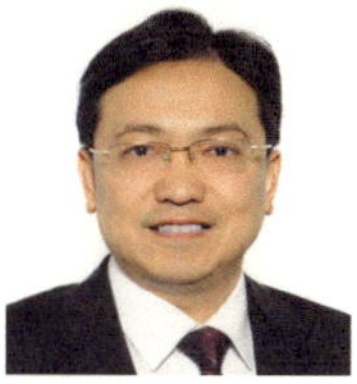

Qiang Yan, MD, FACS, is the vice president of Huzhou Central Hospital and academic leader of the Department of General Surgery and the Department of Hepatopancreatic and Biliary Surgery, Huzhou Central Hospital, Affiliated Huzhou Hospital, Zhejiang University School of Medicine, Huzhou, China. He is a fellow of the Chinese College of Surgeons and a core member of the Committee of Biliary Surgeons, Committee of Minimal and Non-invasive Surgeons, the Chinese Medical Doctor Association (CMDA), and many other academic associations. He is also an editorial board member of the *Chinese Journal of General Surgery, Liver Cancer, and the Chinese Journal of Clinicians.* He is enrolled in the Zhejiang Province New Century 151 Excellent Talents Program. He has finished advanced studies for hepatobiliary pancreatic surgery at Medical Center, Stanford University and Affiliated Hospital, Regensburg University. He got the certificate of Surgical Leadership Program of Harvard Medical School in September 2019. He has more than thirty publications to his credit.

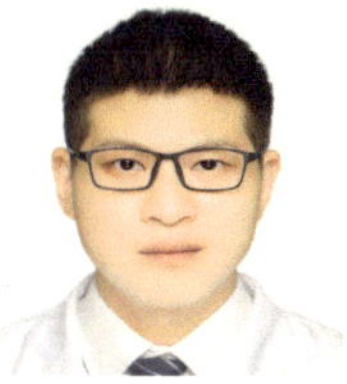

Dr. Zhiping Pan is a medical doctor in the Division of Hepatopancreatic and Biliary (HPB) Surgery, Department of General Surgery, Zhejiang University Huzhou Hospital, China. He is a core member of the hepatobiliary and pancreatic surgery team led by Dr. Qiang Yan. He focuses on the accurate diagnosis and minimally invasive surgical treatment of hepatobiliary and pancreatic diseases.

Contents

Preface **IX**

Section 1
Introduction **1**

Chapter 1 **3**
Introductory Chapter: Biliary Tract – Review and Recent Progress
by Qiang Yan and Zhiping Pan

Section 2
Common Bile Duct Stones **7**

Chapter 2 **9**
Bile Duct Stones
by Diego Rossi Kleinübing, Lailson Alves Rodrigues and Sarah Luiz Brum

Section 3
Choledochal Cyst **23**

Chapter 3 **25**
Choledochal Cyst: Clinical Features, Diagnosis and Treatment Perspectives
by Magaly Torres, Mitzi Becerra, Beatriz Calderón, Iván Salinas, María Ruiz and Jorge Ventura

Chapter 4 **45**
Characteristics, Diagnosis and Treatment of Choledochal Cysts
by Umut Tüysüz

Section 4
Gallbladder Cancer **63**

Chapter 5 **65**
Gallbladder Cancer: Diagnosis and Surgical Management
by Asmita Chopra and Alessandro Paniccia

Section 5
Bile Duct Injury 83

Chapter 6 85
Iatrogenic Biliary Injury Surgical Management
by Alex Zendel and Yaniv Fenig

Preface

Biliary system diseases are a common pathology in medical practice. The biliary tree is characterized by bile duct branches at multiple levels, with innumerable variations present in each branch, giving rise to an increasing geometric progression of biliary anatomy types. Therefore, as an organ, the biliary tract has a certain complexity in the occurrence and development of its disease. The management of biliary tract disease remains a challenging and emerging area of investigation.

This book discusses the natural history, clinical presentation, diagnosis, and medical and surgical management strategies of the varying pathologies that make up biliary diseases such as common bile duct stones (CBDS), choledochal cyst (CC), gallbladder cancer (GBCa), and bile duct injury (BDI). CBDS is a chronic recurrent hepatobiliary disorder that can trigger serious complications, including obstructive jaundice, acute suppurative cholangitis, and acute pancreatitis. Early diagnosis and prompt treatment are the most important factors in managing CBDS. CC, also known as congenital bile duct dilatation, presents with extrahepatic bile duct dilatation. In patients with jaundice, abdominal pain, and a palpable abdominal mass, physicians must have a high clinical suspicion of CC. The biggest challenge in the surgical management is how to ensure the long-term patency of the postoperative biliary system and prevent subsequent strictures, stones and carcinogenesis. GBCa is the most common cancer of the biliary system and has a very poor prognosis when diagnosed at a late stage. Cancer may also present with mild, vague symptoms such as loss of appetite, chronic abdominal discomfort, weight loss, pruritus, scleral icterus, and jaundice. The diagnosis of GBCa is based on a combination of multiple dimensions including history, physical examination, imaging, or biopsy. The treatment of GBCa remains difficult at present. There are few cases amenable to surgical resection, and it again has a low response rate to most adjuvant therapies. BDI is a very feared complication after gallbladder surgery. It occurs because the biliary tract and its blood supply cannot be avoided during dissection. Its most common symptoms are persistent abdominal pain, bloating, nausea and/or vomiting, fever, and jaundice. While its different injury types and degrees determine different surgical repair modalities.

This book is designed to help clinicians better understand and treat biliary system diseases.

Qiang Yan and Zhiping Pan
Department of General Surgery,
Huzhou Central Hospital,
Hu Zhou, China

Section 1

Introduction

Chapter 1

Introductory Chapter: Biliary Tract – Review and Recent Progress

Qiang Yan and Zhiping Pan

1. Introduction

1.1 Biliary diseases

Biliary diseases are common digestive system disorders in clinical practice worldwide. Diseases in this segment of the biliary tract are diverse and can manifest with mild clinical signs or can be life-threatening. These diseases exert their effects on our normal lives and have an impact on our physical well-being. It is important to correctly recognize the features of these disorders and, with the right management options in hand. It presents a challenge for every clinician. This book discusses the work-up, diagnosis, and management of the varying pathologies that make up biliary disease including common bile duct stones (CBDS), choledochal cyst (CC), gallbladder cancer (GBCa), and bile duct injury (BDI). Therefore, it can provide clinicians with a platform to learn about these disorders in order to better serve patients.

2. Chronic recurrent hepatobiliary disease

CBDS is a chronic recurrent hepatobiliary disease whose pathological bases are impaired cholesterol, bilirubin, and bile acid metabolism. The incidence of cholelithiasis is 5% to 15%, in the incidence of CBDS is about 5–30% [1]. This is also associated with serious complications, including obstructive jaundice, acute suppurative cholangitis, and acute pancreatitis. Early diagnosis and prompt treatment are the most important for managing CBDS [2]. Endoscopic ultrasonography (EUS) and magnetic resonance cholangiopancreatography (MRCP) have high sensitivity, specificity, and accuracy for the diagnosis of CBDS. At present, it is recommended that patients with CBDS be treated with minimally invasive surgery promptly after diagnosis to reduce iatrogenic trauma or complications caused by surgery based on expelling the stones. The endoscopic retrograde cholangiopancreatography (ERCP) and laparoscopic transcystic common bile duct exploration (LTCBDE) approaches have become two different minimally invasive treatments for choledocholithiasis [3]. Their advantages of good curative effect, small trauma, quick recovery, and fewer complications have been recognized by the majority of medical workers.

3. Congenital biliary dilation

CC, also known as congenital biliary dilation, presents as the dilation of extrahepatic bile ducts. It has a worldwide incidence of about 1:100,000 to 1:150,000 but the incidence can be as high as 1 in 1000 in Asians [4]. Todani classification focuses on the location and morphology of the lesions and classifies intrahepatic and extrahepatic dilated bile ducts into five types, which are currently the most widely used. CC is a rare anomaly that is sometimes considered a precancerous lesion, which often poses a diagnostic dilemma. The typical presentation of this condition is nonspecific. The medical team must have a high level of clinical suspicion for choledochal cysts when investigating patients with jaundice, abdominal pain, and palpable abdominal masses. Because of these symptoms and the ambiguity of the physical findings, appropriate imaging studies are essential for their diagnosis [5]. The three major principles of surgical management of CC are total cyst resection, resolution of stenosis, and biliopancreatic diversion. The bilio jejunal Roux-en-Y anastomosis is currently the standard surgical procedure for biliary reconstruction. The biggest challenge in the surgical management of biliary cysts is how to ensure long-term postoperative biliary system patency and prevent subsequent strictures, stones, and carcinogenesis. This requires the physician to build systematic thinking preoperatively about the complex conditions and anatomic features that bile duct cysts may combine to properly and meticulously address key intraoperative details.

4. GBCa

GBCa is the most common cancer of the biliary tract system and is ranked as the top six in general gastrointestinal tract neoplasms worldwide [6]. Due to the aggressive behavior and limited treatment options available for GBCa, the prognosis is very poor at late diagnosis. Early detection at a curable stage remains challenging because patients rarely manifest symptoms; indeed, most GBCs are discovered incidentally following cholecystectomy for symptomatic gallbladder stones. Cancer can also present with subtle, vague symptoms such as loss of appetite, chronic abdominal discomfort, weight loss, pruritus, scleral icterus, and jaundice. The diagnosis of GBCa is based on a combination of history, physical examination, laboratory tests, radiological imaging (ultrasound, CT, MRI, and/or PET), and biopsy. Long-standing chronic inflammation is an important driver of GBC, regardless of the lithiasic or non-lithiasic origin. Advances in omics technologies have led to a greater understanding of GBC pathogenesis, revealing mechanisms associated with inflammation-driven tumorigenesis and progression. Surgical resection is the only curative treatment for GBC, but cases suitable for resection are rare and response rates to most adjuvant therapies are very low. Several unmet clinical needs require to be addressed to improve GBC management, including the discovery and validation of reliable biomarkers for screening, treatment selection, and prognosis [7].

5. BDI

BDI is still a much-feared complication following gallbladder surgery. It occurs because of the inability to avoid the biliary tract and its blood supply during dissection. Several factors are associated with an increased risk of BDI associated with cholecystectomy. These include the inability to clearly identify the cystic duct prior to clipping or dividing, surgery for acute cholecystitis, the presence of choledocholithiasis, anatomic variations in the anatomy of the biliary tree, and emergency surgery [8]. The most common complaints of BDI patients are persistent abdominal pain, abdominal distension, nausea and/or vomiting, fever, and jaundice [9]. The clinical manifestations of BDI are related to the type of injury. The two most common clinical conditions are biliary leakage and biliary obstruction. Strasberg classification of BDI is fairly comprehensive for defining the type and extent of injury and guiding surgical repair. The effective surgical management of low-grade Strasberg types A-D injuries can include biliary drainage, primary repair of the bile duct, or duct-to-duct biliary reconstruction. High-grade Strasberg type E injuries should be always repaired with Roux-en-Y hepatojejunostomy [10].

This book covers the above four common diseases of the biliary tract. A focused and concise introduction to the basic concepts, clinical manifestations, diagnosis, and therapeutic measures of each disease is given. It is hoped that this book will help physicians at large to reinforce their personal experience and standardize the behavior of clinical diagnosis and treatment of biliary-related diseases, becoming a powerful helper for front-line clinical workers.

Author details

Qiang Yan[1,2,3,4,5,6]* and Zhiping Pan[1,2,3,4,5,6]

1 Affiliated Huzhou Hospital, Zhejiang University School of Medicine, Huzhou, Zhejiang, China

2 Department of General Surgery, Affiliated Huzhou Hospital, Zhejiang University School of Medicine, Huzhou, Zhejiang, China

3 Department of General Surgery, Affiliated Huzhou Central Hospital, Huzhou University School of Medicine, Huzhou, Zhejiang, China

4 Department of General Surgery, Zhejiang Chinese Medical University, The Fifth School of Clinical Medicine, Huzhou, Zhejiang, China

5 Huzhou Key Laboratory of Intelligent and Digital Precision Surgery, Huzhou, Zhejiang, China

6 Department of General Surgery, Huzhou Central Hospital, Huzhou Key Laboratory of Intelligent and Digital Precision Surgery, Huzhou, Zhejiang, China

*Address all correspondence to: yanqiangdoc@hotmail.com

References

[1] Deng F, Zhou M, Liu PP, et al. Causes associated with recurrent choledocholithiasis following therapeutic endoscopic retrograde cholangiopancreatography: A large sample sized retrospective study. World Journal of Clinical Cases. 2019;**7**(9):1028-1037

[2] Wu Y, Xu CJ, Xu SF. Advances in risk factors for recurrence of common bile duct stones. International Journal of Medical Sciences. 2021;**18**(4):1067-1074

[3] Zhang R, Liu J, Li H, Zeng Q, Wu S, Tian H. Evaluation of therapeutic efficacy, safety and economy of ERCP and LTCBDE in the treatment of common bile duct stones. Frontiers in Physiology. 2022;**13**:949452

[4] Ye Y, Lui VCH, Tam PKH. Pathogenesis of choledochal cyst: Insights from genomics and transcriptomics. Genes (Basel). 2022;**13**(6):1030

[5] Hoilat GJ, John S. Choledochal Cyst. Treasure Island (FL): StatPearls Publishing; 2022

[6] Song X, Hu Y, Li Y, et al. Overview of current targeted therapy in gallbladder cancer. Signal Transduction and Targeted Therapy. 2020;**5**(1):230

[7] Roa JC, García P, Kapoor VK, et al. Gallbladder cancer. Natural Review in Diseases Primers. 2022;**8**(1):69. DOI: 10.1038/s41572-022-00398-y

[8] Ahmad DS, Faulx A. Management of postcholecystectomy biliary complications: A narrative review. The American Journal of Gastroenterology. 2020;**115**(8):1191-1198

[9] Mercado MA, Domínguez I. Classification and management of bile duct injuries. World Journal of Gastrointestinal Surgery. 2011;**3**(4):43-48

[10] de Angelis N, Catena F, Memeo R, et al. 2020 WSES guidelines for the detection and management of bile duct injury during cholecystectomy. World Journal of Emergency Surgery. 2021;**16**(1):30

Section 2

Common Bile Duct Stones

Chapter 2

Bile Duct Stones

Diego Rossi Kleinübing, Lailson Alves Rodrigues and Sarah Luiz Brum

Abstract

Common bile duct stones (CBDS) incidence is about 10–15%. Clinical signs and symptoms are nonspecific but when associated with biochemical tests and abdominal ultrasound, patients can be categorized into low, intermediate, and high risk of choledocholithiasis. These clinical, biochemical, and radiological predictors will direct the diagnostic approach through cholangio magnetic resonance, endoscopic ultrasound, laparoscopic ultrasound, or intraoperative cholangiography. Treatment options must consider technological availability, technical skills, stone size, and bile duct diameter. In general, it involves endoscopic retrograde cholangiopancreatography or surgery for CBDS clearance. For difficult stones, endoscopic sphincterotomy followed by large balloon dilation, mechanical lithotripsy, cholangioscopy-guided lithotripsy, and extracorporeal shock wave lithotripsy are described, mainly as a bridge procedure.

Keywords: gallbladder stones, choledocholithiasis, bile duct stones predictors, bile duct stone diagnosis, bile duct stones treatment

1. Introduction

Gallbladder stone disease has an overall prevalence of approximately 15%. Choledocholithiasis is present in about 10–20% of patients with symptomatic cholelithiasis [1–5]. Secondary choledocholithiasis remains the leading cause of common bile duct stones (CBDS), originating from migration of gallbladder stones into hepatocholedochal duct, while primary choledocholithiasis is a rare cause, mainly affecting the eastern population [4, 6].

The pathophysiology of secondary CBDS is the same as for gallbladder stones. Most gallstones are composed of cholesterol, due to the supersaturation of the bile, leading microcrystals formation. These cholesterol crystals, incorporated into vesicular mucin and associated with bile stasis, form gallstones. While 80–90% are cholesterol gallstones, primary choledocholitiasis is related to brown stones, whose formation occurs directly in the common bile duct (CBD), resulting from mechanical obstruction of bile flow, leading to stasis with subsequent bacterial colonization. However, sometimes there is no obstructive factor, such as bile duct stricture or papillary stenosis. Therefore, dilated CBD, especially after cholecystectomy, is an important factor for primary CBDS [7–9].

Due to the multifactorial etiology of gallbladder stones, CBDS predominates in female gender aged over 55 years, with dietary, genetic, and hormonal associated factors, as metabolic syndrome, obesity, rapid weight loss, family history, pregnancy, multiparity, and oral contraceptives [4, 7, 8].

Symptomatology is quite varied, ranging from completely asymptomatic patients to classic clinical manifestations of biliary lithiasis, such as epigastric or right upper abdominal pain, nausea and vomiting, to obstructive symptoms as fluctuant jaundice, choluria, and acholia. Eventually, patients may present with other complications of choledocholithiasis, for example, acute pancreatitis or cholangitis [6, 10].

Recurrent primary choledocholithiasis is a chronic pathology conceptually characterized by recurrence of common bile duct stones after, at least, 6 months of cholecystectomy. Some risk factors are bile duct greater than 13–15 mm in diameter and with angle smaller than 145°, presence of periampullary diverticulum, biliary stricture or papilla stenosis, and identification of two or more stones in bile duct [3, 11–13].

There are specific predictors of choledocholithiasis, which include clinical findings (obstructive jaundice, acute pancreatitis, or cholangitis), abnormal hepatogram, and presence of a choledochal stone or bile duct dilatation >8 mm [3, 4]. Based on this, patients are stratified in low, intermediate, or high risk of choledocholithiasis which will guide all diagnostic effort and, therefore, treatment approach [1, 2, 6, 14].

2. Diagnosis

Clinical manifestations of choledocholithiasis are nonspecific such as epigastric or upper abdominal pain, nausea, vomiting, and fluctuating jaundice. History of acute pancreatitis, cholangitis, and jaundice are suggestive of choledocholithiasis, since nearly 50% of acute biliary pancreatitis and most cholangitis are caused by stones in the common bile duct (CBD) [6, 15].

Screening for choledocholithiasis includes clinical, biochemical (gamma-glutamyl transpeptidase (GGT), alkaline phosphatase (AF), alanine aminotransferase (ALT), aspartate aminotransferase (AST), and bilirubin) and ultrasound showing CBD greater than 6 mm. These predictors, when normal, have high power to rule out the presence of choledocholithiasis, considering their negative predictive value is greater than 97% [5].

The initial evaluation with predictive factors allows us to stratify patients into high, intermediate, and low probability of choledocholithiasis. These factors are clinical evidence of acute cholangitis, bilirubin greater than 1.7 mg/dL, visualization of common bile duct stone, and dilated CBD on abdominal ultrasound. When two of these factors are present, the probability of choledocholithiasis is high, whereas with normal common bile duct diameter without cholangitis, the probability is low. Patients between these two spectra are stratified as having intermediate probability for diagnosis [3].

Based on the initial screening assessment, when the suspicion of choledocholithiasis is low, laparoscopic cholecystectomy (LC) is recommended. If it is intermediate, the options are endoscopic ultrasound (EUS), magnetic resonance cholangiopancreatography, or even computed tomography (CT scan) in the preoperative period, according to local availability. During intraoperative suspect, laparoscopic ultrasound (LUS) or intraoperative cholangiography (IOC) is indicated [3, 11].

2.1 Abdominal ultrasound

Ultrasound consists of an inexpensive, noninvasive, and widely available method; however, it is operator-dependent with limitations in obese patients in the investigation of choledocholithiasis. The most important contribution is to demonstrate

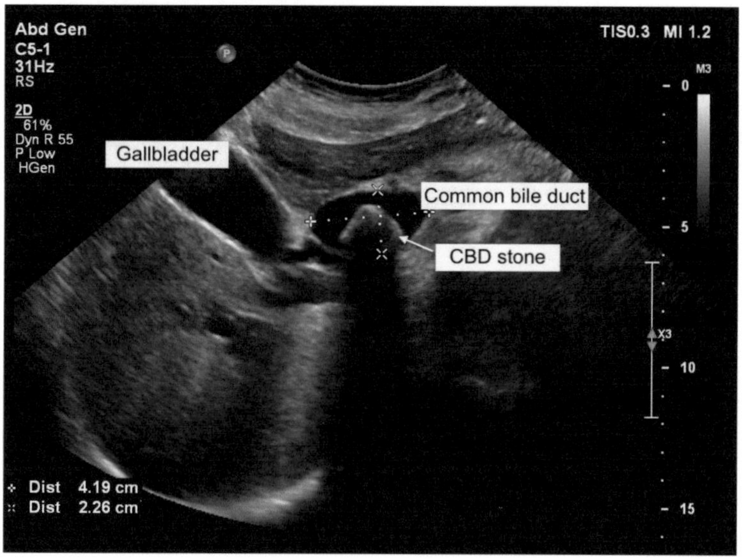

Figure 1.
Ultrasound showing common bile duct dilated (2.28×4.19 cm) with a 2.2 cm stone.

dilation of the CBD above 6 mm at the time of initial screening, although its normality does not exclude the diagnosis [3, 6, 11, 16]. The sensitivity is 73% and specificity is 91% [11]. As we can see in **Figure 1,** the common bile duct is located over the portal vein and the common bile duct stone typically produces posterior acoustic shadow.

2.2 Magnetic resonance cholangiopancreatography

It is recommended in cases of intermediate suspicion of choledocholithiasis, that is, patients with altered biochemical tests, aged >55 years and dilatation of the common bile duct on ultrasound [4], consisting of a noninvasive option, with sensitivity >90% and specificity close to 100%. This accuracy is reduced for stones smaller than 3 mm. It is normally required for the diagnosis of choledocholithiasis before endoscopic intervention or surgical exploration [2].

It suggests choledocholithiasis on T2 when evidence of fluid (bile) as a bright, high-intensity signal on images. Solid material may be suggested by the filling failure—hypointense and well delimited—within the common bile duct, as we see in **Figure 2** [6].

It is contraindicated in patients with claustrophobia, obesity, cardiac pacemakers, or metal clips [3, 4].

2.3 Endoscopic and laparoscopic ultrasound

Endoscopic ultrasound (EUS) is a diagnostic method based on the introduction of an endoscope with an ultrasound transducer into the duodenal bulb, with specificity about 90% and sensitivity of 97% for CBD stones detection [4]. It is indicated mainly for patients who cannot perform magnetic resonance cholangiopancreatography (MRCP), that is, those who have intracranial metallic clips, pacemakers, mechanical heart valves, claustrophobia, and morbid obesity. Its main disadvantage is related to invasiveness, need for anesthetic sedation, and reduced availability. In addition, EUS

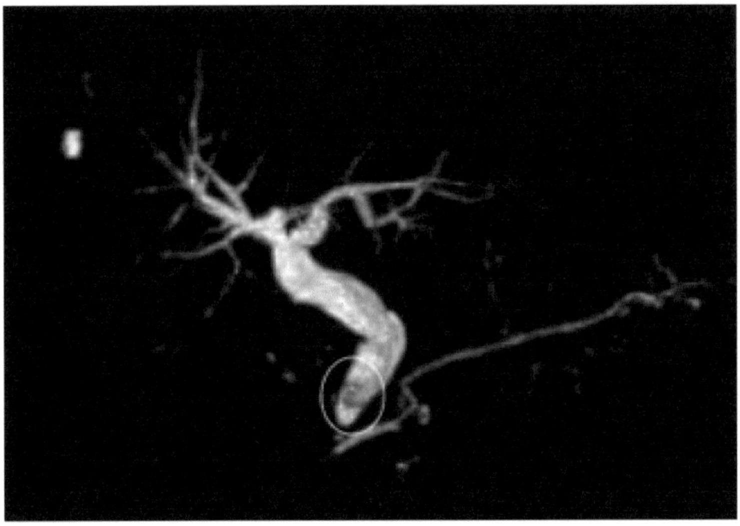

Figure 2.
MRCP showing common bile duct dilated (1.3 cm in diameter) with 0.6 cm stone at distal portion (circle).

is operator-dependent, which also makes it more expensive. Patients with gastric bypass present an important limitation of this method [4, 11].

Laparoscopic ultrasound consists in a specific laparoscopic probe used directly over the common bile duct and is indicated for patients with intermediate risk during intraoperative period which has not been detected by initial investigation by MRCP or EUS [3, 6]. With sensibility estimated in 95% and specificity near 100% [17], its main limitation is proximal biliary tree stone evaluation [18].

The stones are suggested by hyperechoic foci with posterior acoustic shadowing [6].

2.4 Endoscopic retrograde cholangiopancreatography (ERCP)

Method performed by combining upper digestive endoscopy and fluoroscopy presents sensitivity around 82% and specificity near 90% for the CBDS diagnosis. Main disadvantages of this method are invasiveness and risk of pancreatitis in 5–10% of patients. Currently, endoscopic retrograde cholangiopancreatography (ERCP) has been reserved for therapeutic purposes for patients diagnosed with choledocholithiasis by MRCP, endoscopic ultrasound, or even computed tomography [3, 6].

2.5 Computed tomography (CT scan)

Although not routinely used, this method is indicated when the hypotheses of common bile duct stones and a tendency to malignancy coexist or in absence of ERCP or MRCP. Its sensitivity is 78% and specificity is 96%, with reduced accuracy if CBDS <5 mm or bile-like density [6, 11].

There is an option for diagnosing choledocholithiasis with contrast-enhanced CT cholangiography, but contrast is poorly available [6].

As a disadvantage, contrast injection and exposure to ionizing radiation are described [6]. In **Figure 3,** we can see the stone in a patient with right upper abdominal pain and fluctuant jaundice.

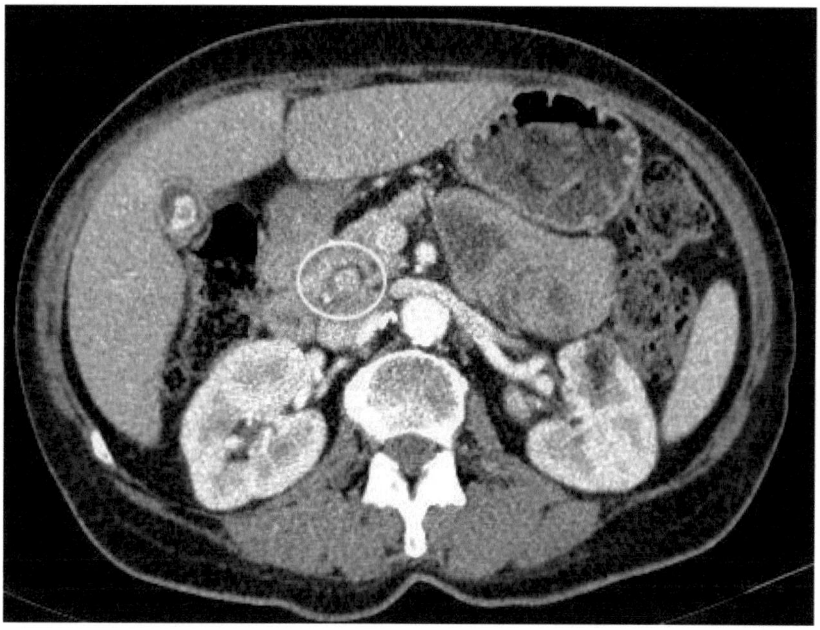

Figure 3.
CT scan showing distal bile duct stone (white circle).

2.6 Intraoperative cholangiography (IOC)

It consists in a useful method to delineate the anatomy of the biliary tree and to demonstrate the presence of intraoperative common bile duct stones. It exhibits sensitivity of 75–99% and specificity around 90–100% for the diagnosis of choledocholithiasis, especially when correlated with clinical, biochemical, and ultrasound findings [2, 5].

IOC can be selectively indicated in patients at high risk of choledocholithiasis undergoing cholecystectomy (history of jaundice, cholangitis or pancreatitis, abnormal biochemical tests, and a CBD > 8 mm in the US) or routinely in all consecutive patients candidates to cholecystectomy, irrespective the risk of CBDS. However, the selective or routine indication remains controversial in the literature. Currently, as we can see in **Figure 4**, IOC is still considered the gold standard for intraoperative biliary anatomy evaluation [4, 5, 19].

3. Treatment

The management of choledocholithiasis is based on bile duct clearance and cholecystectomy, as most ductal stones migrate from gallbladder. Therefore, all patients with common bile duct stones, symptomatic or not, should be managed with gallbladder removal to treat the cause and to avoid recurrence of this chronic hepatobiliary pathology [1, 3, 6].

The approach of the CBDS depends on local technological resources availability, technical skills, moment of diagnosis, stone size, and common bile duct diameter [2, 3].

The treatment of choledocholithiasis involves, in general aspects, ERCP or surgical exploration of the common bile duct, laparoscopic, or open [1, 6]. Therefore, in

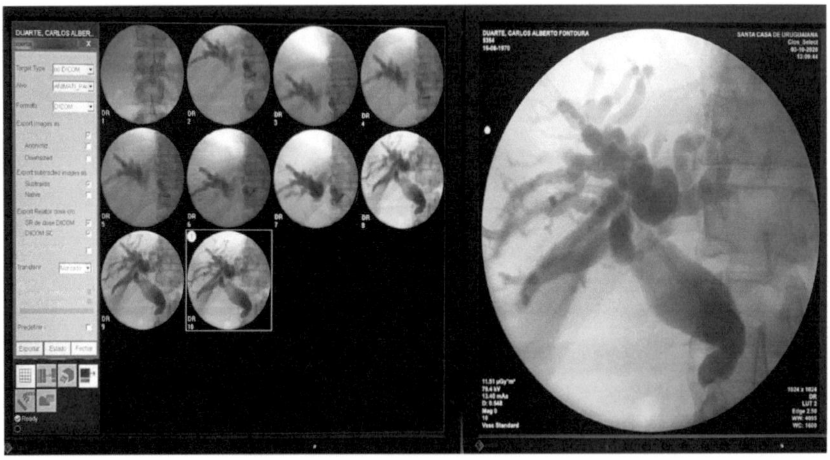

Figure 4.
Intraoperative cholangiography showing intra and extrahepatic bile duct dilation.

non-cholecystectomy patients with choledocholithiasis, CBDS smaller than 1 cm and bile duct with diameter until 1.5 cm, preoperative ERCP followed by laparoscopic cholecystectomy is preferred. In case of unavailable ERCP, the option is to proceed with intraoperative cholangiography, bile duct exploration, and cholecystectomy in a unique procedure, laparoscopic, or open approach. When diagnosis is confirmed intraoperatively by cholangiography or LUS, it is possible to proceed with intraoperative ERCP or surgical exploration in the same surgical act, depending on the surgeon's experience, biliary anatomy, and available resources. Another possibility is to proceed with postoperative ERCP [3]. Finally, in cholecystectomy patients, postoperative ERCP is the gold standard therapy [1, 3, 6]. We emphasize that stone size greater than 1.5 cm and CBD diameter greater than 1.5 cm, if considered isolated or together, are predictors of higher rates of success by surgical exploration than ERCP.

There are no differences in the success rates of gallstone removal regarding pre-, intra-, or postoperative ERCP, which is estimated around 80–90%. However, intraoperative ERCP has lower complication rates and faster hospital discharge. Ideally, as it is performed in a unique time, intraoperative approach is quite advantageous, but the dynamics, resources, and necessary structure are major disadvantages of this strategy [1]. Despite the high success rates in clearance of choledocholithiasis, ERCP presents risks and complications, especially post-ERCP pancreatitis, followed by infection, bleeding, and perforation of the bile ducts. Although there is no definitive consensus, there is a general preference for preoperative ERCP, due to the assurance that there is no more distal obstruction, reducing the need for another intervention [2]. Besides, an interval of up to 2 weeks after ERCP is recommended to proceed with LC [1, 11].

In stones larger than 1.5 cm, endoscopic sphincterotomy followed by large balloon dilation (12–20 mm), mechanical lithotripsy, cholangioscopy-guided lithotripsy, and extracorporeal shock wave lithotripsy are described, mainly as a bridge procedure to definitive ERCP or surgical approach. However, it must be emphasized that this size of stone is normally followed by bile duct dilation, which needs necessarily be considered when one chooses the treatment options [1, 4, 6, 11].

Therefore, stones larger than 1.5 cm, multiple bile duct stones (>15), tortuous biliary anatomy, and a CBD diameter > 2 cm present difficulty of endoscopic and laparoscopic removal, being predictors of open procedure, which will probably evolve associated biliodigestive derivation, preferably choledochojejunostomy Roux-en-Y derivation, to avoid biliary stasis and consequently recurrent choledocholithiasis. Choledochojejunostomy is preferred over choledochoduodenostomy due to lower rates of stone recurrence and complications such as sump syndrome **Figure 5** [1–4, 6, 11, 20–24].

The main complications of surgical treatment are biliary leak at choledochotomy suture or at bile duct-enteric anastomosis, biloma, common bile duct stenosis which may cause also recurrent choledocholithiasis, pancreatic or bile duct injury due to instrumentation, and recurrent ascendent cholangitis mainly with choledochoduodenostomy technique [21, 23–25].

Bile leaks are prevented following general principles of anastomosis as tension-free and well-perfused anastomotic stumps, biliary, and enteric. It is also the crucial anatomical knowledge of common bile duct axial vascularization when performing choledochotomy, which must be longitudinal to avoid vascular section, for bile duct exploration and stones removal. Additionally, one must be certified of the absence of distal bile duct obstruction before proceeding with choledochotomy suture. The occurrence of biliary leak, despite all these precautions, has benign behavior and closes spontaneously in most cases when drain-oriented placed intraoperatively or after biloma percutaneous drainage [26, 27].

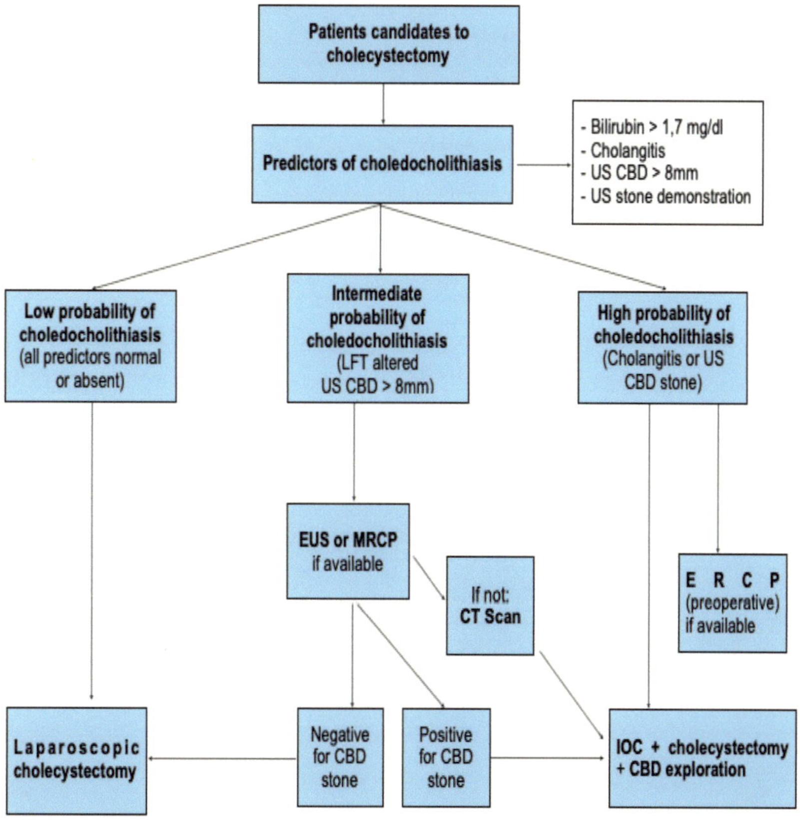

Figure 5.
Diagnosis approach of common bile duct stones flowchart. US: ultrasound, CBD: common bile duct, LFT: liver function tests, EUS: endoscopic ultrasound, MRCP: magnetic resonance cholangiopancreatography, CT Scan: computed tomography, IOC: intraoperative cholangiography, ERCP: endoscopic retrograde cholangiopancreatography.

Biliary strictures are preferably managed through ERCP or transhepatic dilation, depending on the height of bile duct stricture and the magnitude of stenosis. Surgical management with redo anastomosis, a difficult procedure considering previous manipulation, is reserved when endoscopic or percutaneous approach fails [26–29].

The preference for hepatic or choledochojejunostomy is recommended to avoid recurrent ascendent cholangitis also known as sump syndrome [24, 27].

New perspectives, mainly minimally invasive, for bile duct stones treatment include cholangioscopy-guided lithotripsy, extracorporeal shock wave lithotripsy, and laser lithotripsy under direct visualization through ureteroscopes or choledochoscopes employment [30]. SpyGlass™ system is a new device for high-resolution cholangioscopy which may be combined with electrohydraulic lithotripsy during ERCP or with laser lithotripsy, specially applied for difficult bile duct stones [31].

Although not yet widely available and clearly established by the guidelines, all these techniques could be used as adjunct to ERCP or laparoscopic bile duct exploration in order to improve one-step resolution rates in case of simultaneous gallbladder

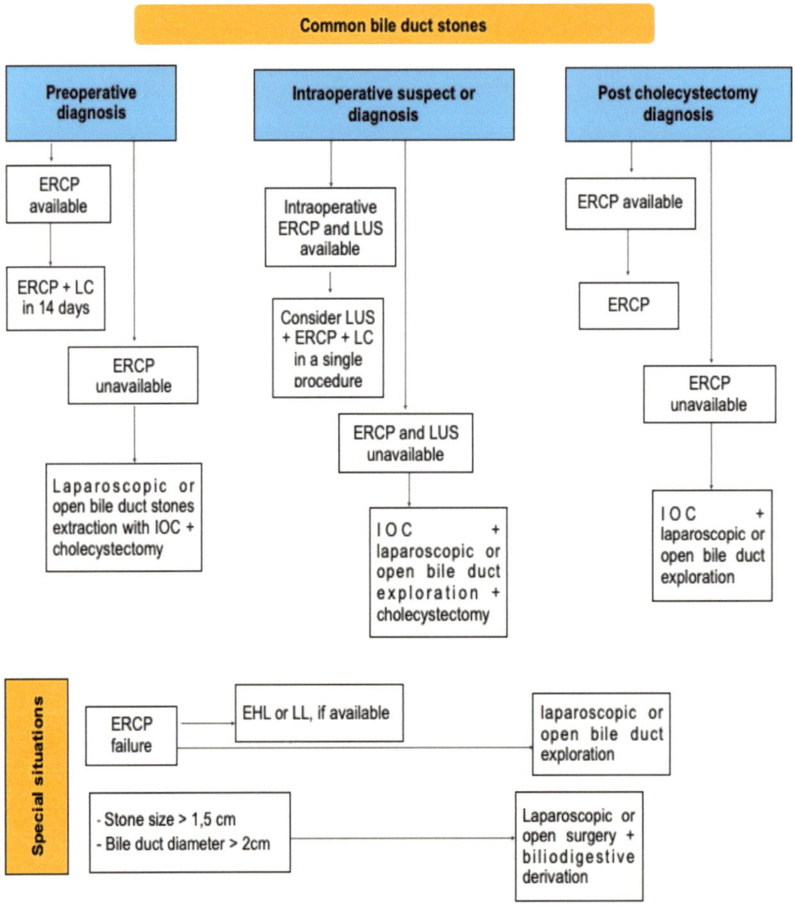

Figure 6.
Management of common bile duct stones flowchart. ERCP: endoscopic retrograde cholangiopancreatography, LC: laparoscopic cholecystectomy, IOC: intraoperative cholangiography, LUS: laparoscopic ultrasound, EHL: cholangioscopy-guided electrohydraulic lithotripsy, LL: laser lithotripsy.

stones or common bile duct clearance if residual choledocholithiasis, according to technical skills development [3, 4, 11, 30, 31].

The summary of management is summarized in **Figure 6**.

4. Conclusions

Bile duct stones is relatively prevalent condition. In patients with gallbladder, the diagnostic effort must include both silent and suspected stone based on clinical, biochemical, and radiological predictors of choledocholithiasis, in the cholecystectomy preoperative period. Once stratified as intermediate or high risk, the investigation will proceed according to local resources availability, preferably with MRCP and ERCP, respectively. The treatment will depend on several factors to be considered, such as the moment of diagnosis, stone size and number, bile duct diameter, ERCP availability, and technical skills. Considering all these factors, the surgeon must propose the best available approach to your patient.

Acknowledgements

We wish to express our gratitude to Santa Casa de Caridade de Uruguaiana, Brazil, where our medical care develops.

We would like to thank Universidade Federal do Pampa, Uruguaiana, Brazil, where our research, teaching, and learning activities develop.

Conflict of interest

The authors declare no conflict of interest.

Abbreviations

AF	alkaline phosphatase
ALT	alanine aminotransferase
AST	aspartate aminotransferase
CBD	common bile duct
CBDS	common bile duct stones
CT	computed tomography
ERCP	endoscopic retrograde cholangiopancreatography
EUS	endoscopic ultrasonography
LUS	laparoscopic ultrasonography
GGT	gamma-glutamyl transpeptidase
IOC	intraoperative cholangiography
LC	laparoscopic cholecystectomy
MRCP	magnetic resonance cholangiopancreatography

Author details

Diego Rossi Kleinübing[1,2]*, Lailson Alves Rodrigues[1] and Sarah Luiz Brum[1]

1 Federal University of Pampa, Uruguaiana, Brazil

2 Hepatobiliary Surgery, HSCU, Uruguaiana, Brazil

*Address all correspondence to: diegokleinubing@unipampa.edu.br

References

[1] Tazuma S, Unno M, Igarashi Y, Inui K, Uchiyama K, Kai M, et al. Evidence-based clinical practice guidelines for cholelithiasis 2016. Journal of Gastroenterology. 2017;**52**(3):276-300

[2] Dasari BVM, Tan CJ, Gurusamy KS, Martin DJ, Kirk G, McKie L, et al. Surgical versus endoscopic treatment of bile duct stones. Cochrane Database of Systematic Reviews. 2013;(12) Art. No.: CD003327. DOI: 10.1002/14651858.CD003327.pub4

[3] Narula VK, Fung EC, Overby DW, Richardson W, Stefanidis D. Clinical spotlight review for the management of choledocholithiasis. Surgical Endoscopy. 2020;**34**(4):1482-1491

[4] Buxbaum J, Fehmi S, Sultan S, Fishman D, Qumseya B, Cortessis V, et al. ASGE guideline on the role of endoscopy in the evaluation and management of choledocholithiasis. Gastrointestinal Endoscopy. 2019;**89**:1075-1105

[5] Kleinubing DR, Riera R, Matos D, Linhares MM. Selective versus routine intraoperative cholangiography for cholecystectomy. Cochrane Database of Systematic Reviews. 2018, 2022;(2) Art. No.: CD012971. DOI: 10.1002/14651858. CD012971. Accessed 15 June

[6] Williams E, Beckingham I, El Sayed G, Gurusamy K, Sturgess R, Webster G, et al. Updated guideline on the management of common bile duct stones (CBDS). Gut. 2017;**66**(5):765-782

[7] Attasaranya S, Fogel E, Lehman G. Choledocholithiasis, ascending cholangitis, and gallstone pancreatitis. Medical Clinics of North America. 2008;**92**:925-960

[8] Wilkins T, Agabin E, Varghese J, Talukder A. Gallbladder dysfunction: Cholecystitis, choledocholithiasis, cholangitis, and biliary dyskinesia. Primary Care Clinics in Office Practice. Dec 2017;**44**(4):575-597. DOI: 10.1016/j.pop.2017.07.002. Epub 2017 Oct 5. PMID: 29132521

[9] Saharia P, Zuidema G, Cameron J. Primary common duct stones. Presented at the Annual Meeting of the Southern Surgical Association. 1976. pp. 5-8

[10] Chae MK, Lee SH, Joo KR. Assessment of the possible risk factors for primary common bile duct stone recurrence after cholecystectomy. Surgical Endoscopy. 2020;**35**(12):6497-6504

[11] Manes G, Paspatis G, Aabakken L, Anderloni A, Arvanitakis M, Ah-Soune P, et al. Endoscopic management of common bile duct stones: European Society of Gastrointestinal Endoscopy (ESGE) guideline. Endoscopy. 2019;**51**(05):472-491

[12] van Dijk AH, de Reuver PR, BesselinkMG, van Laarhoven KJ, Harrison EM, Wigmore SJ, et al. Assessment of available evidence in the management of gallbladder and bile duct stones: A systematic review of international guidelines. HPB. 2017;**19**(4):297-309

[13] Yoo ES, Yoo BM, Kim JH, Hwang JC, Yang MJ, Lee KM, et al. Evaluation of risk factors for recurrent primary common bile duct stone in patients with cholecystectomy. Scandinavian Journal of Gastroenterology. 2018;**53**(4):466-470

[14] Wu Y, Xu CJ, Xu SF. Advances in risk factors for recurrence of common bile duct stones. International Journal of Medical Sciences. 2021;**18**(4):1067-1074

[15] Sperna Weiland CJ, Busch CB, Bhalla A, Bruno MJ, Fockens P, et al.

Performance of diagnostic tools for acute cholangitis in patients with suspected biliary obstruction. Journal of Hepato-Biliary-Pancreatic Sciences. 2022;**29**(4):479-486

[16] Horrow MM. Ultrasound of the extrahepatic bile duct: Issues of size. Ultrasound Quarterly. 2010;**26**(2):67-74

[17] Donoghue S, Jones RM, Bush A, Srinivas G, Bowling K, Andrews S. Cost effectiveness of intraoperative laparoscopic ultrasound for suspected choledocholithiasis; outcomes from a specialist benign upper gastrointestinal unit. The Annals of The Royal College of Surgeons of England. 2020;**102**(8):598-600

[18] Atstupens K, Mukans M, Plaudis H, Pupelis G. The Role of laparoscopic ultrasonography in the evaluation of suspected choledocholithiasis. A single-center experience. Medicina (Kaunas). 2020;**56**(5):246

[19] de Araujo TB, Jotz GP, Zaki CH, Mantelli RA, Fernandes VF, Pretto GG, et al. Intraoperative cholangiography with filling defects: comparative complication analysis of postoperative transcystic duct (TCD) catheter maintenance. Surgical Endoscopy. 2021;**35**(12):6438-6448

[20] Râmboiu S, Ghita F, Raluca-Elena N, Gororgescu I. The role of biliodigestive derivations in the tratment of choledocholithiasis. Current Health Sciences Journal. 2011;**37**(4):181-184

[21] Shojaiefard A, Esmaeilzadeh M, Ghafouri A, Mehrabi A. Various techniques for the surgical treatment of common bile duct stones: A meta review. Gastroenterology Research Practice. 2009:1-12. DOI: 10.1155/2009/840208. Epub 2009 Aug 6. PMID: 19672460; PMCID: PMC2722154

[22] Park CY, Choi SH, Kwon CI, Cho JH, Jang SI, Lee TH, et al. What is the better surgical treatment option for recurrent common bile duct stones? Annals of Surgical Treatment and Research. 2020;**99**(6):329-336

[23] Abraham H, Thomas S, Srivastava A. Sump syndrome: A rare long-term complicationofcholedochoduodenostomy. Case Reports in Gastroenterology. 2017;**11**(2):428-433

[24] Cho CS, D'Angelica MI. Bile duct exploration and biliary-enteric anastomosis. In: Jarnagin WR, editor. Blumgart's Surgery of the Liver, Biliary Tract, and Pancreas. Vol. 5th. Philadelphia: Elsevier Saunders; 2012

[25] Moore MD, McIntyre CA, Eachempati S. Management of complications from biliary surgery. In: Moore L, Todd S, editors. Common Problems in Acute Care Surgery. Springer Cham; 7 Dec 2016. DOI: 10.1007/978-3-319-42792-8. eBook ISBN 978-3-319-42792-8

[26] Anderson CD, Scoggins CR, Chari RS. Reoperative Hepatobiliary Surgery. In: Callery MP, editor. Handbook of Reoperative General Surgery. Malden: Blackwell Publishing Inc.; 2006. pp. 1-16

[27] Kim JY, Kim KW, Ahn C, Hwang S, Lee Y, Shin YM, et al. Spectrum of biliary and nonbiliary complications after laparoscopic cholecystectomy: Radiologic findings. American Journal of Roentgenology. 2008;**191**:783-789

[28] Bismuth H, Majno PE. Biliary strictures: Classification based on the principles of surgical treatment. World Journal of Surgery. 2001;**25**:1241-1244

[29] Strasberg SM, Hawkins W. Reconstruction of the bile duct:

Anatomic principles and surgical techniques. In: Fisher JE, Bland KI, editors. Mastery of Surgery. 5th ed. Philadelphia: Lippincott Williams & Wilkins; 2007. pp. 1128-1144

[30] Bosley ME, Zamora IJ, Neff LP. Choledocholithiasis—A new clinical pathway. Translational Gastroenterology and Hepatology. 2021;**6**:35

[31] Liu YJWQ. Efficacy and safety of SpyGlass system combined with electrohydraulic lithotripsy during endoscopic retrograde cholangiopancreatography in treatment of difficult common bile duct stones. Journal of Clinical Hepatology. 2021;**37**(7):1644-1647

Section 3

Choledochal Cyst

Chapter 3

Choledochal Cyst: Clinical Features, Diagnosis and Treatment Perspectives

Magaly Torres, Mitzi Becerra, Beatriz Calderón, Iván Salinas, María Ruiz and Jorge Ventura

Abstract

Choledochal cyst is a congenital or acquired anomaly affecting the biliary tree in which exists a dilatation of the bile duct, not only the choledochus is affected but also the intrahepatic and extrahepatic ducts might be affected. The clinical presentation is not specific, even the classic triad with abdominal pain, mass, and jaundice is not common as suspected, found only in 10% of cases. Clinicians must rely on imaging studies for diagnosis and classification. The treatment is cyst excision with hepaticoenterostomy in most of the cases, but in some others, a liver transplant would be necessary. These patients require lifelong follow-up due to its rate of recurrence compared with general population.

Keywords: choledochal cyst, biliary cyst, biliary tree, biliary tract disease, jaundice, roux-en-Y, hepaticoenterostomy, hepaticojejunostomy, hepaticoduodenostomy

1. Introduction

Choledochal cyst (CC) is an entity where there is a dilatation at any level of the bile duct, more common in the choledochus, hence its name. Although in almost all the literature, it is referred to as a "choledochal cyst," the most appropriate way to

Age (years)	Range (mm)
≤ 4	2–4
4–6	2–4
6–10	2–6
10–12	3–6
12–14	3–7

Adapted from Witcombe JB, Cremin BJ. The width of the common bile duct in childhood. Pediatr Radiol. 1978;7:147–149.

Table 1.
Mean common bile duct diameter and range according to patient age.

refer to this pathology would be dilation of the bile duct, since it does not necessarily present as a cyst, and it is not necessary to appear in the choledochus either.

Therefore, to refer to a dilated duct, it is necessary to know the normal diameter of the common bile duct (choledochus). A study by Pina and colleagues reports an average of 5–6 mm in diameter of the common bile duct in adult patients; however the diameter varies according to age and measurement method (**Table 1**) [1, 2]. Another study where measurements were made on 173 children aged between 1 day and 13 years reported an average diameter of the common bile duct of 1.27 mm (± 3.3 mm) and < 1.2 mm in newborn and children up to 3 months [3]. Consequently, any measurement greater than reported can be considered abnormal.

2. Classification of choledochal cyst

Diverse classifications have been proposed to categorize the CC. Currently, Todani's classification has been the most extensively accepted (**Figure 1**). It was

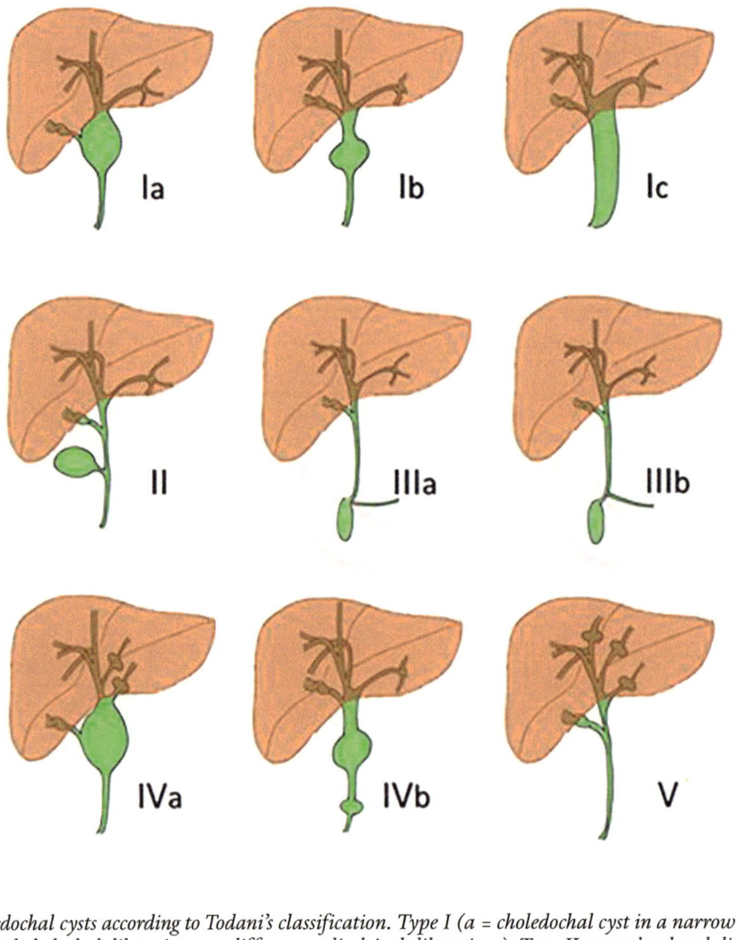

Figure 1.
Types of choledochal cysts according to Todani's classification. Type I (a = choledochal cyst in a narrow sense; b = segmental choledochal dilatation; c = diffuse or cylindrical dilatation.). Type II supraduodenal diverticulum. Type III (a = choledochocele; b = diverticular choledochocele). Type IV multiple dilatations [a = involving the intrahepatic biliary tract; b = sparing the intrahepatic biliary tract. Type V (or Caroli's disease): Corresponds to multiple intrahepatic dilatations.

described in 1977, based on evidence of the existence of various anatomical forms of biliary cystic dilatation that occur not only in the choledochus, but also in any part of the bile duct between the liver and the duodenum, previously the classifications for this entity include only choledochus dilations [4].

According to Todani's classification, CCs are classified into five types:

- Type I: Common type, represents 50–80% of CCs. It is characterized by cystic dilation of the common bile duct. It is further divided into three subgroups: a. choledochal cyst in a narrow sense; b. segmental choledochal dilatation; and c. diffuse or cylindrical dilatation.

- Type II: Diverticulum type in the whole extrahepatic duct, represents 2%.

- Type III: Choledochocele, represents 1.4%–4.5% of CCs. It is an intraduodenal cystic dilation of the distal common bile duct.

- Type IV: Represents 15–35% of CCs. It is further divided into two subgroups. a. Multiple cysts at the intra- and extrahepatic ducts; b. multiple cysts at the extrahepatic duct only.

- Type V: Intrahepatic bile duct cyst (single or multiple). Also known as Caroli's disease, represents 20% of CCs [5].

Furthermore, there exists a special variant of CC named "forme fruste," where the patients present with typical symptoms of CCs and are associated with abnormal pancreaticobiliary duct junction but little or no dilation of biliary ducts. It could be considered as an incomplete or atypical pathology [6].

3. Epidemiology and incidence

There is an outstanding regional tendency, which affects predominantly Asian population with an incidence of 1 in 1000 live births, and two-thirds of the reported cases occur in Japan, compared with an incidence of 1 in 100,000–150,000 live births in the Western population [7, 8].

CCs type I and IV are more common and have a female-to-male ratio of 4:1 or 3:1. The cause for the Asian and female predominance remains under study, recent research studies settle that congenic bile duct dilatation has genetic basis, not only genetically heterogeneous but also non-monogenic, requiring mutations in more than one gene for the disease to develop. That is consistent with the low frequency and sporadic presentation of CC [9–11].

4. Etiology and pathophysiology

The etiology of a choledochal cyst remains unknown at present time, leading to the postulation of multiple theories. "Long common channel" theory by Babbit has been the most accepted explanation for the origin of the choledochal cyst. This theory states that the pancreaticobiliary junction is located outside the duodenal wall [12, 13].

In normal conditions, the common bile duct and the pancreatic duct enter into the duodenal muscle layer (sphincter of Oddi) and join in the submucosal layer just

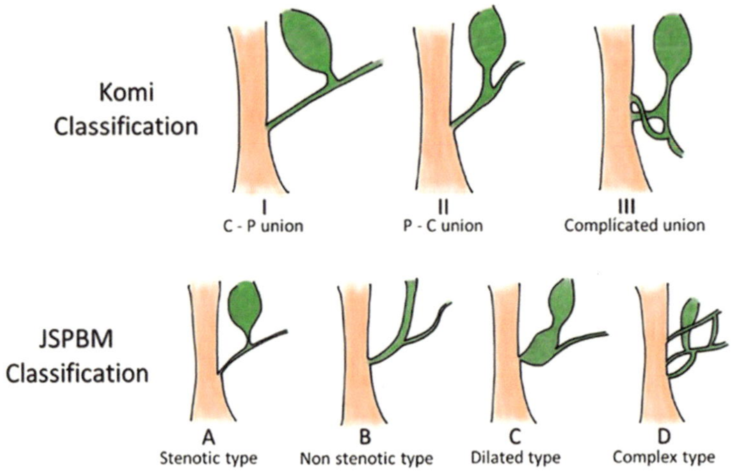

Figure 2.
Pancreaticobiliary maljunction classification. Komi classification and Japanese study group on Pancreaticobiliary Maljunction (JSPBM).

before opening into the duodenal lumen. This junction helps to regulate the output of digestive enzymes into the intestinal lumen but in a pancreaticobiliary maljunction (PBM), there is a dysfunction of the sphincter because the duct is external of the duodenal muscle layer, forming an extended common channel, 1–2 cm proximal to the sphincter of Oddi [14].

The maljunction of both ducts occurs during the fifth week of gestation. In normal embryological development, the pancreatic ventral bud fuses side by side with the dorsal bud, and in the sixth week, 180-degree rotation (clockwise) of ventral and choledochal, bud of the pancreas occurs around the duodenum to reach their finale positions [15]. PBM appears to be associated to the malrotation of the ventral bud, as the proximal portion of the hepatic diverticulum extends and the ventral primordium has been displaced away from the duodenum by elongation of the proximal part of the diverticulum.

Histological and immunohistochemical studies have demonstrated that the union of these two buds might occur in an oblique position, producing the formation of a long common channel [14, 16].

PBM was classified by Komi in 1992 into three types, based on the fusion pattern (**Figure 2**):

- Type I: The bile duct joins with the pancreatic duct forming a right angle. It is presented in 35.3% of the cases.

- Type II: It seems that the pancreatic duct connects to the biliary duct in an acute angle. It was seen in 21.6% of the cases.

- Type III in 43.1% of the cases. It is a complicated junction of both ducts [17].

In 2015, the Committee on Diagnostic Criteria of the Japanese Study Group on Pancreaticobiliary Maljunction (JSGPM) proposed a classification into four types [18]:

- Type A (stenotic type): The narrow segment of the distal common bile duct joins the common channel and shows dilatation of the common bile duct.
- Type B (non-stenotic type): The distal common bile duct without any narrow segment joins the common channel. Without dilatation of the common channel.
- Type C (dilated type): The narrow segment of the distal common bile duct joins the common channel, and abrupt dilatation of the common channel is seen.
- Type D (complex type): PBM associated with annular pancreas, pancreas divisum, or other complicated duct systems.

In addition to PBM and a higher pressure of the pancreatic duct, the developed long channel allows reflux of pancreatic juice into the common bile duct. However, it has been found that not all abnormal pancreaticobiliary junctions present dilatation of the bile duct, which could explain only a part of its pathophysiology.

Pancreatic proenzymes also play an important role in the origin of the choledochal cyst, inasmuch as they come into contact with the bile and activate before reaching the duodenum, they generate a state of inflammation, obstruction, increased pressure in the choledochus, and consequently, greater dilation [19]. Furthermore, trypsinogen, when activated into trypsin, modifies a protein called lithostatin in its insoluble form, aggregating and forming protein plugs. These plugs are compacted in the common channel or in the narrow distal part of the cyst, causing pancreatitis or increasing the pressure of the bile duct so much that it sometimes generates biliary perforation.

Pancreaticobiliary reflux and activation of proenzymes generate intermittent symptoms such as abdominal pain, vomiting, jaundice, and increased aminotransferases in children. This fact is confirmed by a retrospective study of 80 patients where biliary amylase measurements were performed, finding a relationship between the presence of biliary amylase and clinical manifestations, with the presence of jaundice as the most common symptom in those with amylase <200 U/L, and with the presence of abdominal pain in those with amylase >200 U/L [20].

It has been observed in adulthood that pancreaticobiliary reflux presents as dilatation of the bile duct and malignancy. This is secondary to the fact that biliary stasis, which was previously mixed with the refluxing pancreatic enzymes, creates damage to the biliary epithelium. Chronic inflammation activates the point mutation of KRAS, overexpresses COX2, and inactivates TP53, generating greater cell proliferation and consequently epithelial hyperplasia, which appears benign in childhood, but in adulthood presents as dysplasia and subsequent carcinogenesis. The site of malignant occurrence is generally within the cyst, but it can be anywhere within the biliary tree [21].

On the other hand, Babbitt's theory is confronted by authors who state that PBM is present in only 50–80% of cases and that in choledochal cyst diagnosed prenatally, there wasn't the presence of reflux, and suggest that neonatal pancreatic acini are not able to produce enough pancreatic enzymes [22]. For unknown reason, despite the presence of PBM, bile duct dilatation may not occur and frequently does not generate symptoms. Therefore, in these patients, PBM tends to be diagnosed at a later stage [23].

This previous theory applies to choledochal cyst types I and IV. Regarding type II (true CBD diverticulum) and type III (choledochocele), it is suspected that the cause is related to biliary duplications cysts for type II and biliary or duodenal duplications cysts for type III [24].

Type V CC and fibrocystic liver disease are related with both being a spectrum of the same congenital disease; ductal dysgenesis affects the biliary tree at multiple levels from the small intrahepatic bile ducts (congenital hepatic fibrosis) to the larger bile ducts (Caroli disease). The etiology type V CC is accepted to be a halt in the remodeling of the ductal plates, and it is associated with biliary atresia [25].

Alternatively, suboptimal number of ganglion cells has been demonstrated in the narrow portion in the distal common bile duct of patients with choledochal cyst when compared with controls. This might lead to the dilation of the proximal segment of the common bile duct, describing a pathogenesis similar to achalasia and Hirschsprung's disease [26].

5. Prenatal diagnosis

The bile duct cyst is scarcely detected in the prenatal stage, the cases reported in the literature range between 20 and 30sdg, being the earliest case described in the 16th week of gestation [27, 28]. The multi-slice high-resolution ultrasound visualizes several planes simultaneously, including sagittal, coronal, transverse, and oblique views being the main tool in the prenatal approach allowing an early diagnosis [27–29].

Among the suggestive findings is the presence of an anechoic cystic image in the right upper quadrant without central vascularity to the application of the Doppler and which is in relation to the contiguity with the gallbladder, in addition to allowing to evaluate the position of the cyst, the state of the proximal ducts, vascular anatomy, and the hepatic echotexture [27, 29].

The advantage of prenatal diagnosis is that it allows the multidisciplinary team adequate neonatal support and prompt surgical planning. During pregnancy, the behavior should be expectant with follow-up ultrasounds, prioritizing childbirth. After birth, the diagnosis can be confirmed with magnetic resonance cholangiopancreatography. There are no international publications so far about perinatal management [30, 31].

Differential diagnosis should include retroperitoneal cysts (hydronephrosis, polycystic kidney, cystic neuroblastoma, or adrenal hematoma) and intraperitoneal cysts (ovarian cysts, epiploic and mesenteric cysts, intestinal duplication, intestinal atresia, biliary atresia, pancreatic and hepatic cysts) [31, 32].

In a series of 13 patients with biliary disease and abnormal prenatal examinations, the correct diagnosis was made prenatally only in 15% of cases. The difficulty in differential diagnosis in the newborn lies between the bile duct cyst and cystic biliary atresia. Given the difficulty that exists of differential between these two entities by prenatal ultrasound, a child with presumed bile duct cyst should undergo an early examination to rule out biliary atresia. So far there are no unequivocal differential parameters that are accepted [30–32].

6. Clinical features

Clinical presentation patterns differ according to the age group at onset of symptoms and the type of cyst. The classic triad of abdominal pain, abdominal mass in the right upper quadrant, and jaundice, although predominant in children, is only reported in 5–10% [33, 34].

Abdominal pain is the most frequent symptom (61–94%) with a slight predominance in older children and adults, which has an intermittent course with a variable time interval from days to years [35, 36]. Abdominal mass and jaundice are usually a manifestation of newborns and infants. Cholangitis, pancreatitis, and liver function test abnormalities are common and are thought to be secondary to a PBM or choledocholithiasis [36–38].

The infantile presentation is characterized by obstructive cholestatic syndrome. Jaundice follows an intermittent pattern since the obstruction of the biliary tree is incomplete; unlike cystic biliary atresia, the main differential diagnosis in this age group.

The presentation of acute abdomen secondary to biliary peritonitis due to rupture of the cyst is rare, predominantly in infants (1–2%). Older children and adults with choledochal cyst present biliary or pancreatic symptoms, mainly associated with abdominal pain. The clinic in this age range is given by entities secondary to chronic biliary stasis, manifesting as complications: cholelithiasis (49%), cholangitis (32%), acute pancreatitis (10%), hepatolithiasis (7%), biliary carcinoma (3%), portal hypertension (2%), and chronic pancreatitis (2%) [39–43]. Fifteen percent of patients with CC may be asymptomatic [36].

On the one hand, some specialized centers in Asia reported direct comparison studies about the clinicopathological differences between children and adults with choledochal cyst. Pediatric patients were more likely to have abdominal mass (52.4% vs. 21.2%) and jaundice (33.3 vs. 0%) compared with adults. Children are more frequently associated with PBM (85.7% vs. 59.6%) and sudden severe stenosis of the terminal common bile duct (76.2% vs. 42.3%). Adults were more likely to have abdominal pain (98% vs. 76.2%), frequently stone disease, and they are more associated with neoplasms (21.2% vs. 21.0%). Malignancy rates are widely reported to be 14–18% [44–46].

On the other hand, a multi-institutional analysis from eight centers in North America and Europe reported clinical characteristics among children and adults, with mean age at diagnosis of 5 years and 45 years, respectively. Adults had more abdominal pain than children (71.8% vs. 40.7%), and children had more jaundice compared with adults (31.9% vs. 11.6%) [36].

Regarding the symptoms according to the type of cyst, jaundice is observed mainly in type I (56%) and IV cysts. Hepatomegaly, palpable mass and episodes of biliary pancreatitis are more prevalent in type I. Exclusively intrahepatic cysts (type V) present mainly with cholangitis and gallstones [47].

7. Diagnosis

There is no specific marker for choledochal cyst in blood tests, what commonly occur are variations in serum concentrations of amylase, bilirubin, and hepatobiliary enzymes when the patient becomes symptomatic; however, in asymptomatic patients, it can occur or not some variation in blood tests.

Ultrasonography (US) is the initial study when pathology of the bile duct is suspected, the advantage of this study is that it is noninvasive, and in expert hands, it can give a very approximate diagnosis. The main finding in US is dilation of the biliary tract, although it is also useful for evaluating the position of the cyst, the proximal ducts, vascularity, whether there are stones in the bile duct and the characteristics of the liver parenchyma.

A technectium-99 HIDA scan may provide more information if a choledochal cyst is suspected by US, being helpful to distinguish a cyst for biliary atresia.

The abdominal computed tomography (CT) scan can show the bile duct along with intrahepatic and intrapancreatic ducts; it is especially useful to rule out tumors at this level with the disadvantage of exposing the patient to radiation and the difficulty to observe the common channel and the biliopancreatic junction clearly. Therefore, CT cholangiography is more sensitive to assess the biliary tree, it identifies the presence of stones and diagnose the choledochal cyst; with a sensitivity above 90%, but with the risk of generating hepatotoxicity or nephrotoxicity due to the contrast medium [48].

For these reasons, the most recommended study is magnetic resonance cholangiopancreatography (MRCP), which has a sensitivity of 90–100% for diagnosis, with the advantage of not being invasive and not exposing radiation (**Figure 3**). Some centers even have the possibility of generating 3D images for better visualization. This study allows evaluation of the anatomy of the intrahepatic and extrahepatic bile ducts, the pancreaticobiliary junction, as well as the measurement of the length of the common channel, which is generally >15 mm [49–51].

Endoscopic retrograde cholangiopancreatography (ERCP) is also a diagnostic option; however, it is not the most common to perform due to its invasive method, although it is very useful, especially in those patients whose clinical and imaging studies are inconclusive. With this study, the path of the common channel, the common bile duct, and the position of the cyst can be assessed. However, ERCP relies on

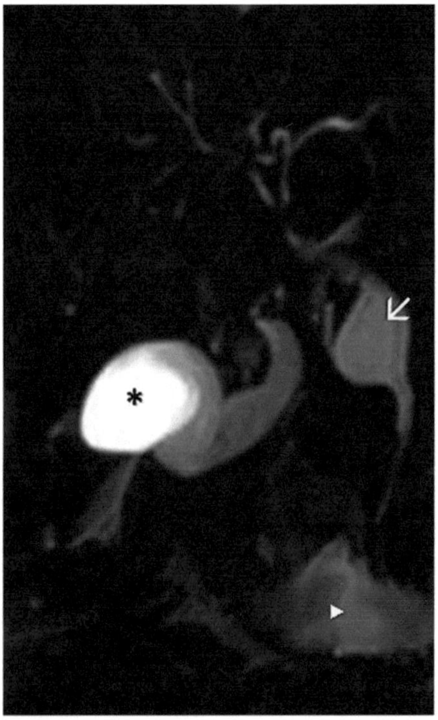

Figure 3.
Coronal T2 MRCP shows a cystic dilation of the common bile duct (arrow) with preserved intrahepatic bile ducts. The gallbladder (asterisk) and the duodenum (arrowhead) are visualized as well.

experienced personnel to perform the procedure, with a 10% rate of complications such as pancreatitis, infection, or bleeding. [52].

Intraoperative cholangiography (IOCG), like ERCP, is not indicated as a routine diagnostic method, it is only suggested in exceptional cases where previous studies have not been conclusive.

8. Management

Medical treatment limits to the administration of antimicrobial therapy in case of cholangitis or supportive therapy in pancreatitis, trying to stabilize the patient prior to operative approach. If rupture of the cyst manifests, a drainage must be placed, pointing out the weirdness of these presentation [53].

Historically, drainage or cystenterostomy was the surgical management, but the high risk of malignant transformation and the recurrence of the symptoms demands aggressive surgical management as the overriding treatment [53, 54].

The prenatal diagnosis of congenital biliary dilatation (CBD) has helped to follow these patients after birth, establishing the ideal time to treat them, if the conditions of the patient allow it, the surgical procedure is recommended at the age of 6 months old. About half of the patients with prenatally diagnosis of CBD are asymptomatic; but if obstructive jaundice, cholangitis, pancreatitis, liver dysfunction, vomiting due to compression of the gastric outlet, or even rupture of the cyst development may be a mandatory earlier surgical exploration, even in the neonatal period [54].

Surgical treatment depends on the CC type. Type I, which is the most common, requires complete cyst excision followed by restoration of the biliary-enteric continuity.

A transverse or oblique incision is the traditional way to reach the hepatic hilum, but the laparoscopic approach (LA) has been increasingly adopted since 1995 when the first successful laparoscopic cyst excision with hepaticojejunostomy (HJ) was performed. A systematic review and update meta-analysis where 1767 patients were enrolled (853 laparoscopic group, 914 open group) reported that the operative time was longer in laparoscopic group, but also less intraoperative bleeding and less intraoperative blood transfusion as well as less time to initial feeding. Length of hospital stay was longer in open group. Short- and long-term postoperative complications were similar in both groups, but the total postoperative morbidity was lower in the laparoscopic group [55].

Minimal invasive robotic-assisted (RA) cyst excision and Roux-en-Y HJ were first reported by Woo in 2006 in a Type I cyst; since then, this practice has gained supporters. In a systematic review and meta-analysis, six studies with 484 patients (307 LA and 177 RA) were analyzed, the results and total complications showed no significant difference between the two groups. [56, 57]. Examination of the data regarding robotic CC excision is needed to determine the utility of this approach in children [53].

The CC transection should be at level of the common hepatic duct to assure a wide anastomosis, a complete excision of the distal portion into the duodenum just above of the pancreatic duct to avoid damage. It is not mandatory to perform IOCG, unless there are no images prior surgery through MRCP; although it is reported that in infants the biliopancreatic junction is very small and can easily go unnoticed during the CC excision. Therefore, if any doubts exist about the situation of the pancreatico-biliary junction, it is recommended to perform IOCG for reducing the risk of injury to the main pancreatic duct.

Some authors practice intraoperative antegrade cholangiography to evaluate also the common channel in all cases because endoscopic retrograde cholangiopancreatography

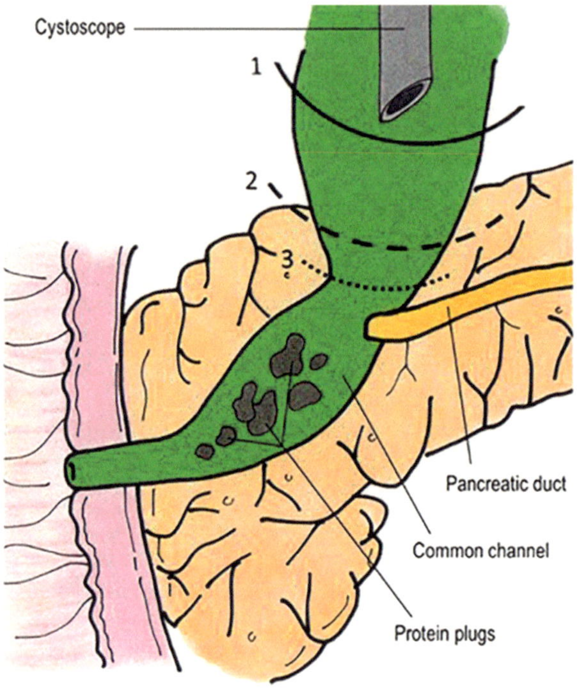

Figure 4.
Intraoperative cystoscopy of the distal portion of the cyst with plug proteins. Level 1 likelihood of leaving residual cyst. Level 2 adequate to perform the transection. Level 3 likelihood of injuring the pancreatic duct.

is difficult to perform in early infancy due to the skill required and the potential for complications.

During the transection of the cyst, an adequate view of the hepatic ducts near the dilation is essential to discard stenosis or hypoplasia, which is related to bad prognosis. If protein plugs are present, wash them out by irrigating with saline solution or remove them with a blunt instrument or a pediatric cystoscope (**Figure 4**) [21, 58].

The biliary reconstruction can be performed through either Roux-en-Y HJ or hepaticoduodenostomy (HD). A systematic review and meta-analysis reported 715 patients, of which 403 (56.3%) were performed a HJ and 312 (43.6%) a HD. Operative time, operative bleeding and length of stay favoring HD, similar rates of complications, including cholangitis. Some disadvantages of the HD are the bile reflux with an estimated incidence of ~5% and require more research and long-term studies [59]. The latest findings in patients followed up by Takada endoscopically demonstrate mild to moderate gastric erosion, but in his study, the development of metaplasia in the stomach [60] is unknown.

A wide Kocher maneuver and a further distal anastomosis in the duodenum have been described to decrease the bile reflux [61]. HD has the advantage to follow through with endoscopic revisions if a late complication is presented, like stenosis of the anastomosis or intrahepatic lithiasis. It is worth to mention that the HD is easier to perform laparoscopically in contrast to the technically challenging HJ. To prevent stenosis of the anastomosis, it is recommended to avoid excessive dissection when dissecting the anterior wall and completely excise ulcerative lesions from the inner wall of the cyst.

A prospective randomized controlled trial describes that a shorter loop Roux-en-Y HJ reconstruction for choledochal cyst is equally effective individualizing the length of the loop based on the distance between the hepatic hilum and the umbilicus, compared with the traditional 40 cm length loop; with no episodes of cholangitis in either group in the following 6 months [62].

8.1 Management for the other choledochal cysts

Type II is a diverticulum of the bile duct, it is the most infrequent presentation of a CC. Surgical removal through laparoscopic approach with excellent results in the reports, but it is known that long-term follow-up and more clinical reports are needed [63].

Type III is a cystic dilatation of the distal common bile duct within the ampulla of Vater protruding into the duodenum, also called choledochocele. The treatment depends on the type of choledochocele, needing endoscopic transduodenal drainage of the lesion in pure choledochocele and with sphincterotomy and complete excision in diverticular choledochocele. Multiple endoscopic technics have been referred such as balloon dilation after incision of the cyst or stent placement, unroofing by partial snare excision of the cyst wall, or complete resection with a polypectomy snare [64, 65].

Type IVa or IVb CC involves dilatation of both intrahepatic and extrahepatic biliary trees. The standard procedure remains to be a complete excision of the dilated common bile duct and a hepaticoenterostomy. Depending on imaging studies, a hepatic segmentectomy or lobectomy might be needed in case of obstruction or to eradicate the segment with the most dilated intrahepatic cysts.

Major late complications such as pancreatic duct stones, intrahepatic calculi, stenosis might need other interventions such as pylorus-preserving pancreatoduodenectomy or duodenum-preserving pancreatic head resection. And sometimes a liver transplant is the only way to preserve a high quality of life [66].

Type V CC benefits from liver transplantation, a related living donor should be considered in time before the onset of life-threatening complications [66, 67].

9. Outcome and complications

The advancement of surgical treatment to include cyst excision has resulted in minimal morbidity and mortality and reduced the number of late complications, compared with past operative treatment of cystenterostomy. The most common short-term outcome in hepaticoenterostomy is anastomotic leakage and as a late complication continues to be anastomotic stricture (2.5–17%) and cholangitis (23–40%) [68–71].

Perioperative morbidity is higher in adults than children (35.1% vs. 16.3%), requiring more surgical procedures following resection of the common bile duct cyst. However, adults were more likely to have wound, hepatobiliary, or gastrointestinal complications: seromas (3.1%), wound infections (9.7%), and perihepatic abscesses (7.7%). Instead, children had more anastomotic leaks (3%) and gastrointestinal tract perforations (3%) [36].

Early diagnosis and cyst excision result in low complication rates in most experienced centers. The technique of Roux-en-Y HJ is favored by most, although comparable results can be achieved by HD. Anyway, either procedure can be performed laparoscopically as well [68, 69]. In most reports comparing laparoscopic cyst excision with open cyst excision in children, operative time was found to be longer and overall costs higher when laparoscopy was used, but there was significantly less blood loss, and the duration of hospitalization was shorter. There were no significant differences in the incidence of bile leakage or wound infection rates. Although technically challenging and time-consuming, laparoscopic excision imparts less surgical stress on patients than open excision, and parents are generally more satisfied with the smaller scars.

Despite late complications being reduced with current surgical management, studies suggest that long-term follow-up is indicated due to the potential for problems such as anastomotic stricture, cholangitis, intrahepatic stone formation, and malignancy [69, 72]. Malignant degeneration occurs more often in type I and IV cysts and rarely in type II and III. This is particularly important in incompletely resected cystic hepatic ducts or recurrent cysts [46, 73].

Biliary cancer is reported in 5–10% of patients, increasing the incidence greater than 50% in patients over 50 years. The risk of malignancy is greatly reduced after cyst excision but is still elevated as compared with the general population, with an incidence ranging between 2.5 and 28% in adults. Nevertheless, it is reduced between 0.7 and 5.4% after complete surgical excision, with a 95.5% 5-year survival (adults 94.6%; children, 97.2%) [36, 74]. Therefore, lifelong follow-up with ultrasound, liver profile, and CA19–9 levels are recommended annually. Some authors perform biochemical follow with aspartate transaminase and alkaline phosphatase, every 4 months for 2 years; then every 6 months for 5 years [46].

A technectium-99 HIDA scan at 6 and 18 months after surgery can reveal mild episodes of cholangitis in asymptomatic patients or in those with occasional symptoms (less than two episodes per year), requiring only conservative therapy. If cholangitis is recurrent, a reoperation is advocated. In addition, technectium-99 HIDA scan can suggest the presence of anastomotic stricture with delayed flow greater than 60 minutes. However, percutaneous transhepatic cholangiography has still been considered to achieve definitive diagnosis [75].

Anastomotic stricture could occur as a consequence of small, tensive anastomosis, inflammation, or infection. Among the most used options are endoscopic retrograde cholangiopancreatography, percutaneous transhepatic biliary drainage, balloon dilation, and stenting with good results. Some authors pointed out that balloon dilation should be the first step as successful rate was 81%, whereas reoperation was considered as the final choice in all circumstances [69, 76].

Intrahepatic stone formation in the intraoperative setting has been evaluated and reported in the literature and seen in patients who showed no stone formation in the preoperative course. Stone formation has been reported to occur anywhere from 3 to 22 years postoperatively. However, if the duct is patent and there is no stenosis of the hepaticojejunostomy, stones are likely to pass spontaneously [77]. Intrahepatic stones usually present in cases of stenosis that initially cause bile stasis and lead to stone formation.

Todani and colleagues reported a 25-year review with the identification of biliary complications primarily associated with either anastomotic stricture or primary ductal stricture and recommended a wide hepatic hilum anastomosis to prevent biliary complications [78].

10. Conclusions

Choledochal cyst is a biliary anomaly that is often diagnosed at early age due to the imaging studies that are currently used. A careful and meticulous search can help establish early treatment, before serious sequelae arise.

Although the management of CC is established with acceptable results, a high rate of complications related to surgical procedures is still reported, so it is necessary to acquire an extensive knowledge of the different variants and provide greater technical skills that are acquired with practice to have better results and minimize the number of complications. In the same way, follow-up is necessary to detect the presence of malignancy in time and offer timely treatment.

Conflict of interest

The authors declare no conflict of interest.

Author details

Magaly Torres*, Mitzi Becerra, Beatriz Calderón, Iván Salinas, María Ruiz and Jorge Ventura
Pediatric Surgery Department, Hospital de Pediatría CMNO IMSS, Guadalajara, México

*Address all correspondence to: magtorresa@gmail.com

References

[1] Witcombe JB, Cremin BJ. The width of the common bile duct in childhood. Pediatric Radiology. 1978;7:147-149

[2] Pina L, Pucci A, Rodríguez A, Novelli D, Urrutia J, Gutiérrez L. Anatomía quirúrgica del conducto colédoco: revisión de la clasificación topográfica. Revista Chilena de Cirugía. 2016;**69**:22-27

[3] Hernanz SM, Ambrosino MM, Freeman PC, Quinn CB. Common bile duct in children: Sonographic dimensions. Radiology. 1995;**195**(1): 193-195

[4] Todani T, Watanabe Y, Narusue M, Tabuchi K, Okajima K. Congenital bile duct cysts: Classification, operative procedures, and review of thirty-seven cases including cancer arising from choledochal cyst. American Journal of Surgery. 1997;**134**:263-269

[5] Singham J, Yoshida EM, Scudamore CH. Choledochal cysts: Part 1 of 3: Classification and pathogenesis. Canadian Journal of Surgery. 2009;**52**(5):434-440

[6] Lilly JR, Stellin GP, Karrer FM. Forme fruste choledochal cyst. Journal of Pediatric Surgery. 1985;**20**:449-451

[7] O'Neill JA. Choledochal cyst. Current Problems in Surgery. 1992;**29**(6):361-410

[8] Moslim MA, Takahashi H, Seifarth FG, Walsh RM, Morris-Stiff G. Choledochal cyst disease in a Western center: A 30-year experience. Journal of Gastrointestinal Surgery. 2016;**20**(8):1453-1463

[9] Liu CL, Fan ST, Lo CM, Lam CM, Poon RT, Wong J. Choledochal cysts in adults. Archives of Surgery. 2002;**137**(4):465-468

[10] Wong JK, Campbell D, Ngo ND, Yeung F, Cheng G, Tang C, et al. Genetic study of congenital bile-duct dilatation identifies de novo and inherited variants in functionally related genes. BMC Medical Genomics. 2016;**9**(1):75

[11] Guo WL, Geng J, Zhao JG, Fang F, Huang SG, Wang J. Gene expression profiling reveals upregulated FUT1 and MYBPC1 in children with pancreaticobiliary maljunction. Brazilian Journal of Medical and Biological Research. 2019;**52**(8):e8522

[12] Hamid R, Bhat NA, Ahmad M, Singh B. Choledochal cyst (CDC). In: Neri V, editor. Gastrointestinal Surgery - New Technical Proposals [Internet]. London: IntechOpen; 2018. DOI: 10.5772/intechopen.72938

[13] Babbitt DP, Starshak RJ, Clemett AR. Choledochal cyst: A concept of etiology. The American Journal of Roentgenology, Radium Therapy, and Nuclear Medicine. 1973;**119**:57-622

[14] Hosomura N, Fujii H. Embryology of Pancreaticobiliary Maljunction. In: Kamisawa T, Ando H, editors. Pancreaticobiliary Maljunction and Congenital Biliary Dilatation. Singapore: Springer; 2018. pp. 11-16

[15] Friedmacher F, Ford KE, Davenport M. Choledochal malformations: Global research, scientific advances and key controversies. Pediatric Surgery International. 2019;**35**:273-282

[16] Le Roy B, Gagnière J, Filaire L, Fontarensky M, Hordonneau C, Buc E.

Pancreaticobiliary maljunction and choledochal cysts: From embryogenesis to therapeutics aspects. Surgical and Radiologic Anatomy. 2016;**38**(9): 1053-1060

[17] Komi N, Takehara H, Kunitomo K, Miyoshi Y, Yagi T. Does the type of anomalous arrangement of pancreaticobiliary ducts influence the surgery and prognosis of choledochal cyst? Journal of Pediatric Surgery. 1992;**27**(6):728-731

[18] Urushihara N, Hamada Y, Kamisawa T, Fujii H, Koshinaga T, Morotomi Y, et al. Classification of pancreaticobiliary maljunction and clinical features in children. Journal of Hepato-Biliary-Pancreatic Sciences. 2017;**24**(8):449-455

[19] Turowski C, Knisely AS, Davenport M. Role of pressure and pancreatic reflux in the aetiology of choledochal malformation. The British Journal of Surgery. 2011;**98**:1319-1326

[20] Jung SM, Seo JM, Lee SK. The relationship between biliary amylase and the clinical features of Choledochal cysts in pediatric patients. World Journal of Surgery. 2012;**36**:2098-2101

[21] Kamisawa T, Kaneko T, Itoi T, Ando H. Pancreaticobiliary maljunction and congenital biliary dilatation. The Lancet Gastroenterology & Hepatology. 2017;**2**:610-618

[22] Imazu M, Iwai N, Tokiwa K, Shimotake T, Kimura O, Ono S. Factors of biliary carcinogenesis in choledochal cysts. European Journal of Pediatric Surgery. 2001;**11**(1):24-27

[23] Morine Y, Shimada M, Takamatsu H, Araida T, Endo I, Kubota M, et al. Clinical features of pancreaticobiliary maljunction: Update analysis of 2nd Japan- nationwide survey. Journal of Hepato-Biliary Pancreatic Sciences. 2013;**20**:472-480

[24] Kagiyama S, Okazaki K, Yamamoto Y, Yamamoto Y. Anatomic variants of choledochocele and manometric measurements of pressure in the cele and the orifice zone. The American Journal of Gastroenterology. 1987;**82**(7):641-649

[25] Levy AD, Rohrmann CA, Murakata LA, Lonergan GJ. Caroli's disease: Radiologic spectrum with pathologic correlation. AJR. American Journal of Roentgenology. 2002;**179**(4):1053-1057

[26] Kusunoki M, Yamamura T, Takahashi T, Kantoh M, Ishikawa Y, Utsunomiya J. Choledochal cyst. Its possible autonomic involvement in the bile duct. Archives of Surgery. 1987;**122**(9):997-1000

[27] Dewbury KC, Aluwihare AP, Birch SJ, Freeman NV. Prenatal ultrasound demonstration of a choledochal cyst. The British Journal of Radiology. 1980;**53**(633):906-907

[28] Todani T, Urushihara N, Morotomi Y, Watanabe Y, Uemura S, Noda T, et al. Characteristics of choledochal cysts in neonates and early infants. European Journal of Pediatric Surgery. 1995;**5**(3):143-145

[29] Lee IH, Kim GJ. Fetal choledochal cyst diagnosed at 22 weeks of gestation by three-dimensional ultrasonography: A case report. Journal of Korean Medical Science. 2008;**23**(5):909-911

[30] Weng R, Hu W, Cai S, Guo X, Luo Q. Prenatal diagnosis and prognosis assessment of congenital choledochal cyst in 21 cases. Journal of Obstetrics and Gynaecology. 2016;**36**(3):324-327

[31] Mackenzie TC, Howell LJ, Flake AW, Adzick NS. The management of prenatally diagnosed choledochal cysts. Journal of Pediatric Surgery. 2001;**36**(8):1241-1243

[32] Chen W, Geng J, Tan YL, Zhao L, Jia HH, Guo WL. Different characteristics of infants diagnosed with congenital choledochal malformation prenatally or postnatally. Scientific Reports. 2021;**11**(1):20

[33] Shah OJ, Shera AH, Zargar SA, et al. Choledochal cysts in children and adults with contrasting profiles: 11-year experience at a tertiary care center in Kashmir. World Journal of Surgery. 2009;**33**:2403-2411

[34] Murphy AJ, Axt JR, Lovvorn HN 3rd. Associations between pediatric choledochal cysts, biliary atresia, and congenital cardiac anomalies. The Journal of Surgical Research. 2012;**177**:59-63

[35] Gadelhak N, Shehta A, Hamed H. Diagnosis and management of chodeochal cyst: 20 years of single center experience. World Journal of Gastroenterology. 2014;**20**(22):7061-7066

[36] Soares KC, Kim Y, Spolverato G, et al. Presentation and clinical outcomes of Choledochal cysts in children and adults: A multi-institutional analysis. JAMA Surgery. 2015;**150**(6):577-584

[37] Swisher SG, Cates JA, Hunt KK, et al. Pancreatitis associated with adult choledochal cysts. Pancreas. 1994;**9**:633-637

[38] Rao KL, Chowdhary SK, Kumar D. Choledochal cyst associated with portal hypertension. Pediatric Surgery International. 2003;**19**:729-732

[39] Yamaguchi M. Congenital choledochal cyst. Analysis of 1,433 patients in the Japanese literature. American Journal of Surgery. 1980;**140**(5):653-657

[40] Ngoc Son T, Thanh Liem N, Manh HV. One-staged or two-staged surgery for perforated choledochal cyst with bile peritonitis in children? A single center experience with 27 cases. Pediatric Surgery International. 2014;**30**(3):287-290

[41] Nicholl M, Pitt HA, Wolf P, et al. Choledochal cysts in western adults: Complexities compared to children. Journal of Gastrointestinal Surgery. 2004;**8**:245-252

[42] Edil BH, Cameron JL, Reddy S, Lum Y, Lipsett PA, Nathan H, et al. Choledochal cyst disease in children and adults: A 30-year single-institution experience. Journal of the American College of Surgeons. 2008;**206**(5):1000-1005

[43] Saluja SS, Nayeem M, Sharma BC, et al. Management of choledochal cysts and their complications. The American Surgeon. 2012;**78**:284-290

[44] Huang CS, Huang CC, Chen DF. Choledochal cysts: Differences between pediatric and adult patients. Journal of Gastrointestinal Surgery. 2010;**14**:1105-1110

[45] Jang SM, Lee BS, Kim KK, Lee JN, Koo YS, Kim YS, et al. Clinical comparison of choledochal cysts between children and adults. Korean J Hepatobiliary Pancreat Surg. Aug 2011;**15**(3):157-163

[46] Wiseman K, Buczkowski AK, Chung SW, Francoeur J, Schaeffer D, Scudamore CH. Epidemiology, presentation, diagnosis, and outcomes of choledochal cysts in adults in an urban environment. American Journal of Surgery. 2005;**189**(5):527-531

[47] De Vries JS, De Vries S, Aronson DC, Bosman DK, Rauws EAJ, Bosma A, et al. Choledochal cysts: Age of presentation, symptoms, and late complications related to Todani's classification. Journal of Pediatric Surgery. 2022;**37**(11):1568-1573

[48] Lam W, Lam TP, Saing H. Cholangiography and CT cholangiography of pediatric patients with choledochal cysts. AJR. American Journal of Roentgenology. 1999;**173**:401-405

[49] Huang CT, Lee HC, Chen WT, Jiang CB, Shih SL, Yeung CY. Usefulness of magnetic resonance cholangiopancreatography in pancreatobiliary abnormalities in pediatric patients. Pediatrics and Neonatology. 2011 Dec;**52**(6):332-336

[50] Park DH, Kim MH, Lee SK, Lee SS, Choi JS, Lee YS, et al. Can MRCP replace the diagnostic role of ERCP for patients with choledochal cysts? Gastrointestinal Endoscopy. 2005;**62**(3):360-366

[51] Wang P, Gong Y, Lu S, Chen J. Three-dimensional visualization technique compared with magnetic resonance cholangiopancreatography for evaluation of anatomic variants of pediatric congenital choledochal cysts. Pediatric Surgery International. 2021;**37**:705-713

[52] Åvitsland TL, Aabakken L. Endoscopic retrograde cholangiopancreatography in infants and children. Endoscopy International Open. 2021;**09**:292-296

[53] Jones RE, Zagory JA, Clark RA, Pandya SR. A narrative review of the modern surgical management of pediatric choledochal cysts. Transl Gastroenterol Hepatol. 2021;**25**(6):37

[54] Okada T, Sasaki F, Ueki S, Hirokata G, Okuyama K, Cho K, et al. Postnatal management for prenatally diagnosed choledochal cysts. Journal of Pediatric Surgery. 2004;**39**(7):1055-1058

[55] Sun R, Zhao N, Zhao K, Su Z, Zhang Y, et al. Comparison of efficacy and safety of laparoscopic excision and open operation in children with choledochal cysts: A systematic review and update meta-analysis. PLoS One. 2020;**15**(9):e0239857

[56] Woo R, Le D, Albanese CT, Kim SS. Robot-assisted laparoscopic resection of a type I choledochal cyst in a child. Journal of Laparoendoscopic Advanced Surgical Techniques. 2006;**16**(2):179-183

[57] Yin T, Chen S, Li Q, Huang T, Li L, Diao M. Comparison of outcomes and safety of laparoscopic and robotic-assisted cyst excision and hepaticojejunostomy for choledochal cysts: A systematic review and meta-analysis. Annals of Medicine and Surgery (Lond). 2022;**75**:103412

[58] Takeshita N, Ota T, Yamamoto M. Forty-year experience with flow-diversion surgery for patients with congenital choledochal cysts with pancreaticobiliary maljunction at a single institution. Annals of Surgery. 2011;**254**(6):1050-1053

[59] Hinojosa-Gonzalez DE, Bueno LC, Roblesgil-Medrano A, Salgado-Garza G, Hurtado-Arellano S, Farias JS, et al. Laparoscopic vs open portoenterostomy in biliary atresia: A systematic review and meta-analysis. Pediatric Surgery International. 2021;**37**(11):1477-1487

[60] Takada K, Hamada Y, Watanabe K, Tanano A, Tokuhara K, Kamiyama Y. Duodenogastric reflux following biliary reconstruction after excision of choledochal cyst. Pediatric Surgery International. 2005;**21**(1):1-4

[61] Santore MT, Behar BJ, Blinman TA, Doolin EJ, Hedrick HL, Mattei P. Hepaticoduodenostomy vs hepaticojejunostomy for reconstruction

after resection of choledochal cyst. Journal of Pediatric Surgery. 2011;**46**(1):209-213

[62] Diao M, Li L, Zhang JZ, Cheng W. A shorter loop in roux-Y hepatojejunostomy reconstruction for choledochal cysts is equally effective: Preliminary results of a prospective randomized study. Journal of Pediatric Surgery. 2010;**45**(4):845-847

[63] Grottesi A, Iacovitti S, Ciano P, Catarci M, Borrini F, Zippi M. Simultaneous laparoscopic removal of a Todani type II choledochal cyst and a microlithiasic cholecystitis. Annals of Hepatobiliary Pancreatic Surgery. 2022. DOI: 10.14701/ahbps.22-011

[64] Law R, Topazian M. Diagnosis and treatment of choledochoceles. Clinical Gastroenterology and Hepatology. 2014;**12**(2):196-203

[65] Itoi T, Gotoda T, Yasuda I, Katanuma A, Ryozawa S, Irisawa A, et al. Balloon-catheter-assisted complete endoscopic snare resection for choledochocele by using double-channel duodenoscope. Gastrointestinal Endoscopy. 2007;**66**(3):622-625

[66] Xia HT, Dong JH, Yang T, Zeng JP, Liang B. Extrahepatic cyst excision and partial hepatectomy for Todani type IV-A cysts. Digestive and Liver Disease. 2014;**46**(11):1025-1030

[67] Lasagni C, Morana F, Strazzabosco. Fibrocystic liver disease: Novel concepts and translational perspectives. Transl. Gastroenterología y Hepatología. 2021;**6**:26

[68] Ndoye NA, Wellé IB, Cissé L, Guèye D, Diouf C, Mbaye PA, et al. Choledochal cyst in children in Dakar: Diagnostic and therapeutic aspects. African Journal of Paediatric Surgery. 2021;**18**(3):168-170

[69] Yeung F, Fung ACH, Chung PHY, Wong KKY. Short-term and long-term outcomes after roux-en-Y hepaticojejunostomy versus hepaticoduodenostomy following laparoscopic excision of choledochal cyst in children. Surgical Endoscopy. 2020;**34**(5):2172-2177

[70] Nguyen HV, Do DH, Nguyen HV, Vu TH, Hong QQ, Vo CT, et al. Treatment of complex complications after choledochal cyst resection by multiple minimal invasive therapies: A case report. International Journal of Surgery Case Reports. 2020;**73**:130-133

[71] Atkinson HD, Fischer CP, de Jong CH, Madhavan KK, Parks RW, Garden OJ. Choledochal cysts in adults and their complications. HPB: The Official Journal of the International Hepato Pancreato Biliary Association. 2003;**5**(2):105-110

[72] Miyano G, Koyama M, Miyake H, Kaneshiro M, Morita K, Nakajima H, et al. Comparison of laparoscopic hepaticojejunostomy and open hepaticojejunostomy. Can stenosis of the hilar hepatic duct affect postoperative outcome? Asian journal of endoscopic. Surgery. 2017;**10**(3):295-300

[73] Ng DW, Chiow AK, Poh WT, Tan SS. Metachronous cholangiocarcinoma 13 years post resection of choledochal cyst-is long-term follow-up useful?: A case study and review of the literature. Surgical Case Report. 2016;**2**(1):60

[74] Yamataka A, Lane GJ, Cazares J. Laparoscopic surgery for biliary atresia and choledochal cyst. Seminars in Pediatric Surgery. 2012;**21**(3):201-210

[75] Adhikari DFM, D, Mehta HB, Olino K, Riall TS, Brown KM. Incidence of hepaticojejunostomy stricture after hepaticojejunostomy. Surgery. 2016;**160**(3):691-698

[76] Belli G, Rotondano G, D'Agostino A, Iannelli A, Marano I, Santangelo ML. Cystic dilation of extrahepatic bile ducts in adulthood: Diagnosis, surgical treatment and long-term results. HPB Surgery. 1998;**10**(6):379-384

[77] Yamataka A, Segawa O, Kobayashi H, Kato Y, Miyano T. Intraoperative pancreatoscopy for pancreatic duct stone debris distal to the common channel in choledochal cyst. Journal of Pediatric Surgery. 2000;**35**(1):1-4

[78] Todani T, Watanabe Y, Urushihara N, Noda T, Morotomi Y. Biliary complications after excisional procedure for choledochal cyst. Journal of Pediatric Surgery. 1995;**30**(3):478-481

Chapter 4

Characteristics, Diagnosis and Treatment of Choledochal Cysts

Umut Tüysüz

Abstract

Choledochal cysts are congenital dilatations of the intra- and extrahepatic biliary tract that cause various pancreatic and hepatobiliary disorders. Pancreaticobiliary maljunction (PBM) results in choledochal cysts. PBM is a congenital pancreatic and bile duct juncture anomaly. It is widely accepted that the clinical presence of PBM is an etiological factor in the pathogenesis of biliary carcinogenesis in patients with choledochal cysts. For definitive diagnosis, ultrasonography sometimes shows the relationship with the biliary tract. If USG findings cannot rule out other causes, ideally MRI should be performed together with MRCP. CT may be the initial test for undiagnosed common bile duct malformations. In rare cases where conventional imaging results are uncertain, nuclear hepatobiliary iminodiacetic acid (HIDA) scanning enables the evaluation of radiological trace of involvement and accumulation in cystic structures associated with the biliary system. Todani added five anomalies and organized the most commonly used classification system. There are five subtypes. A type I cyst, A choledochal diverticulum (Todani type II), Choledochoceles (Todani type III), type IV cyst, Caroli disease (Todani type V). Surgical treatment should be based on the extent of biliary involvement based on the widely used Todani classification and anatomical findings and the presence or absence of PBM. The standard treatment in most CCs is the resection of the bile duct up to the lobar bifurcation. Residual postoperative intrapancreatic choledochal cyst may also lead to secondary carcinogenesis and associated morbidity. The localization of the pancreatic cyst is inside the head of the pancreas, close to the neck and to the left of the bile duct. Surgical treatment options include laparoscopic treatment. Its main advantages include excellent visualization and low blood loss.

Keywords: choledochal cysts, pancreaticobiliary maljunction, choledochal diverticulum, choledochoceles, caroli disease, cholangiocarcinoma

1. Introduction

Choledochal cysts are congenital dilatations of the intra- and extrahepatic biliary tract that cause various pancreatic and hepatobiliary disorders, collectively known as congenital cystic dilatation of the common bile duct [1]. Its total incidence is about 1/100,000–1/150,000 in the Western population and 1/1000 in the Asian population [2]. The male-to-female ratio was reported to be approximately 1:3 or 1:4 [3]. Since they do not contain an epithelial structure, they are not real cysts. They are choledochal malformations that can be detected by imaging and cover various morphological anomalies of the biliary ductal system [4–6]. The exact cause of choledochal malformations is unclear. However, a number of theories were proposed about their pathogenesis, ranging from complete congenital anomaly to sequelae of multiorgan disease process [2]. Choledochal malformations are prone to complications such as cholestasis, pancreatitis, cholangitis, and cholelithiasis. Moreover, some of them, especially those associated with chronic inflammation, have a 50% higher probability of malignant transformation [2]. Choledochal malformations are mostly observed in the pediatric population. An estimated 25% of them are detected in the first year of life and after, while 35–55% by the age of 10 [2]. Up to 20% of them occur in adulthood and have a worse prognosis than in childhood [7, 8].

The similar incidence rates of choledochal cysts in the Western and Eastern cohorts are probably associated with similar etiology. Babbitt's theory is the most commonly proposed one. According to this theory, pancreaticobiliary maljunction (PBM) results in choledochal cysts. PBM is a congenital pancreatic and bile duct juncture anomaly caused by the union of the common duct and pancreatic and bile ducts outside the wall of the duodenum [9]. It is widely accepted that the clinical presence of PBM is an etiological factor in the pathogenesis of biliary carcinogenesis in patients with choledochal cysts. Here, the pancreatic duct and the bile duct are united at a position 1–2 cm proximal to the sphincter of Oddi [10–14]. The presence of pancreaticobiliary ductus junction anomaly allows reflux of pancreatic secretions into the biliary tree. This is the accepted theory for etiopathogenesis of cysts [15, 16]. The clinical presence of PBM is widely considered to be etiological in biliary carcinogenesis in patients with choledochal cysts [17–20]. PBM induces the reflux of pancreatic enzymes into the bile duct, which is thought to be involved in the formation of the bile duct cysts and the development of cancer within the biliary cyst [21]. Biliary cysts (BDC) have a 100–1000 times lower incidence rates in Western series [22–24]. Most of the studies with Western series reported BDC in adults, which had less association with PBM compared with Eastern series [25]. The common duct theory posits that the PBM above the sphincter of Oddi complex causes reflux of pancreatic and digestive enzymes into the bile duct. As a result, wall weakness and subsequent dilatation occur. Moreover, high levels of phospholipase A2 and trypsinogen in the bile of choledochal cyst patients were suggested to exacerbate inflammation and epithelial deterioration in the bile duct [26].

There is no consensus for the diagnosis of PBM, at least in Western countries. Diagnosis includes MRCP, ERCP, and functional criteria (measurement of intrabiliary amylase level). The diagnosis of PBM is based on two strict criteria: (1) The presence of conclusive evidence for the intraduodenal junction between the choledochal and the main pancreatic duct, and (2) the presence of an abnormal common duct longer than 10 mm. PBM is found in only 50–80% of choledochal cyst cases [27].

In a multicenter study conducted in France, 72.2% of patients with BDC were found to have PBM. While 66.8% of the patients were adults, 33.2% were children (<15 years old). The most common symptoms were abdominal pain (64.3%), jaundice (24.7%), cholangitis (24%), and pancreatitis (23.6%). At the same time, the most common types were C-P type I (57.2%), P-C type II (34.5%), and type III (complex type) (8.3%). The mean common duct length was 15.8–6.8 mm while children had shorter common ducts (5.3–13.8 mm). The common duct was longer than 6 mm in 97.6% of the patients and longer than 10 mm in 90.5%. Considering the abnormal common duct longer than 8 mm based on the diagnosis, the sensitivity and specificity rates were 97.6% and 80%, respectively, while the positive and negative predictive values were 99.2% and 57.1%, respectively. In the same study, the coexistence of the common duct longer than 8 mm and amylase values above 8000 UI/L were associated with positive predictive and specificity rates of more than 90%. In terms of the association between PBM and Todani BDC types, there was a coexistence rate of 78.4% for type I and IVb, 16.6% for type II, 33.3% for type III, and 19% for type IVa. Although the relationship between type IV and type I BDC and PBM was not significant, the incidence of biliary cancer in type I and type IV patients with PBM was 83.3 and 25%, respectively. The relationship between PBM and BDC is similar in Asia and the West cohorts as 72% [22, 23]. Likewise, coexistence of PBM is more frequent in type IV and type I (69 and 78%, respectively), which is less in type II and III (16.6 and 33.3%, respectively) [9, 22–25]. However, there was no association between type V (Caroli disease) and PBM [28]. PBM type P-C subtype is more commonly found with BDC-type Ic (fusiform) while PBM-type C-P subtype is more common with BDC-type Ia. Therefore, in patients with slightly large choledochal (approximately 20 mm), the evidence of the presence of P-C-type PBM represents a key indication for the diagnosis of Todani BDC type Ic diagnosis. Then, complete resection is planned [29, 30]. Anatomical studies showed that 80–85% of adults have a short common duct, whose mean length was reported to be 4.6 mm ± 2.2 mm. In the last study, the mean common duct length was found to be 13.8 ± 5 in patients with suspected PBM. This also confirmed Kawisawa's notion of considering common duct length as the main morphological diagnostic tool for PBM [24]. However, there is no consensus for the cutoff value for the abnormally long common duct. This length is variable during infancy. More than 90% of adults and infants had a common duct length equal to or greater than 10 mm. Taking a cutoff value of 8 mm for the abnormal common duct length may indicate high precision for the diagnosis of PBM. Apart from morphological tools, functional methods using intrabiliary amylase measurement are easy to perform. In one study, intrabiliary mean amylase values were significantly higher in patients with PBM compared with those without PBM (> 50,000 versus <2000, respectively). A literature survey also showed that intrabiliary amylase value of >10,000 UI/L is an important functional tool to confirm the diagnosis of PBM [31]. Intrabiliary amylase concentration can be measured by the following methods: (1) by intraoperative sampling from the gallbladder during cholecystectomy prior to cholangiography or any other manipulation; (2) preoperatively through transhepatic fine-needle aspiration from the gallbladder; and (3) less frequently through bile aspiration during ERCP [32]. In the case of intrabiliary amylase level > 8000 UI/L and common duct length of >8 mm, a definitive diagnosis of PBM can be made with a sensitivity of 87% and a positive predictive value of 90%. However, if the intrabiliary amylase level is normal, the diagnosis of PBM cannot be completely ruled out. When the intrabiliary amylase level is normal and the common duct length is <8 mm, negative predictive value is close to 90%. Therefore, this could be an appropriate method to rule out PBM and then BDC diagnosis. Likewise, the level of amylase in the gallbladder is slightly higher than in the biliary tract, which may support the stagnation theory in carcinogenesis. These theories blamed pancreatic fluid reflux and its attack to biliary tract as the main culprit of cancer degeneration in especially dilated segments against the cholangiocarcinoma degeneration in the distal part of the biliary tree even when these observations were not directly related to Caroli disease, with or without PBM. In the presence of PBM, especially the Todani type I BDC, the incidence of biliary cancer seems to increase. Cholangiocarcinoma cancer degeneration develops 10 years earlier than those without PBM [33]. There is a high risk of cancer degeneration in patients who underwent cyst enterostomy due to BDC [34, 35]. The global cancer incidence of 8.3% in patients with PBM also including children observed in a Western cohort study was similar to what was reported in Eastern series, albeit at a slightly higher rate [22, 23].

Each entity has different imaging findings, diagnostic features, and surgical management. When it is not detected incidentally in prenatal imaging, it is frequently found in the right upper quadrant ultrasound examination performed for the symptoms and signs of pain, palpable mass, or cholestasis in childhood and young adults [2, 36]. Bile duct larger than 10 mm without obstruction in childhood is always associated with choledochal malformation [37]. For definitive diagnosis, ultrasonography sometimes shows the relationship with the biliary tract. If USG findings cannot rule out other causes, ideally MRI should be performed together with MRCP [36]. The T2-weighted technique routinely used in MRCP allows for a quality depiction of the hepatobiliary system [9]. MRI-MRCP with or without contrast enhancement is a method of choice in preoperative planning. Contrast application indicates malignant change and the choice of alternative approach [38]. CT may be the initial test for undiagnosed common bile duct malformations that are detected later in life or incidentally. The frequency of incidentally detected choledochal cysts in adults has increased from 10–36% due to the availability and convenience of CT [7]. The sensitivity of CT cholangiopancreatography in showing the common pancreatobiliary and pancreatic duct is 64% [39]. Due to concomitant sedation requirements, ERCP and percutaneous cholangiography carry independent risks and should be reserved for situations that are difficult, complicated, or contraindicated for MRI [40]. Diagnostic confirmation is more difficult in individuals with a cholecystectomy history. MRCP has been used more than ERCP or intraoperative cholangiography in the last 10 years for the diagnosis of PBM. MRCP is the most useful method for detecting PBM as it shows the junction of the common pancreatic duct and the common bile duct outside the duodenal wall even in patients with a clearly normal common duct. In the most recent series, the detection rate of PBM by MRCP is 82–100% [41]. Therefore, in patients with or without BDC, MRCP has been indeed used more frequently as the first-choice method than the endoscopic ultrasound or ERCP for focusing on the pancreatic head region [42]. In rare cases where conventional imaging results are uncertain, nuclear hepatobiliary iminodiacetic acid (HIDA) scanning enables the evaluation of radiological trace of involvement and accumulation in cystic structures associated with the biliary system. This is especially important in distinguishing of true choledochal malformation from imitations such as pancreatic pseudocyst and duodenal duplication cyst [43]. Combining preoperative and intraoperative imaging methods during surgical intervention planning reduces the need for preoperative and postoperative ERCP or percutaneous transhepatic cholangiography. Indeed, the addition of intraoperative cholangiopancreatography to preoperative MRCP, especially in pediatric patients, effectively determines intrahepatic biliary structures. This, in turn, may change surgical planning and diagnostic classification by reducing invasive preoperative imaging methods [44]. Ultrasound, MRI-MRCP with or without contrast enhancement, and CT are considered in evaluating complications and examining malignant transformation.

2. Clinical presentation and diagnosis

In adults, symptoms are usually nonspecific, vague abdominal pain being the most common [15]. When specific symptoms arise, they are typically of acute biliary tract and pancreatic origin [45]. In some patients, the classic symptom triad of abdominal pain, palpable abdominal mass, and jaundice occurs in only 25% of adults, while 85% of children have at least two features of the classic triad. Unexpected presentations such as gastric outlet obstruction, cyst perforation, giant cystolithiasis, giant cyst, and mixed type were reported [46]. Although the frequency of emerging symptoms is similar in Western and Eastern populations, associated biliary conditions such as cholecystitis, cholangitis, and choledocholithiasis are more common at presentation in the Eastern population [20, 22]. Recently, ultrasound has been found to have high sensitivity in the examination of biliary tract diseases [47]. Prenatal diagnosis was also defined in some cases at the 15th week of gestation [48]. In the evaluation of intrapancreatic residual choledochal cyst, it is important that the soft tissue neoplasm is found within the cyst wall, and the wall has a uniform and smooth structure, which should be indicated in the imaging [49]. Peripancreatic lymph nodes are classified as abnormal growth in residual choledochal cysts to prevent carcinogenesis misdiagnosis [50]. In this context, spiral CT-type B has higher resolution than ultrasound and MRCP. All three diagnostic methods can be used together. Serum CA19-9 and carcinoembryonic antigen are listed in the routine preoperative examination of choledochal cyst and are used as important reference indices for the prediction of bile duct carcinogenesis [51]. Caroli syndrome may present with right upper quadrant pain or signs of portal hypertension. It is usually a childhood or young adult disease.

3. Classification of common bile duct malformations

It is important to categorize malformations for the purpose of appropriate management and risk classification. First in 1959, Alonso-Lej proposed a classification scheme that included four anomalies of the biliary tree. Later, in 1977, Todani added five anomalies and organized the most commonly used classification system [33, 52]. In the Todani classification, a type I cyst features fusiform or spherical dilatation in the entire extrahepatic bile duct. It is the most common type in both the Western and Eastern populations. It is observed in 65–84% of the Eastern cohort and 67–73% in the Western cohort. It is divided into three within itself: type Ia: diffuse cystic dilatation, type Ib: focal saccular cystic dilatation, and type Ic: diffuse fusiform dilatation.

Type Ib cystic dilatation typically results from the more distal common choledochal segment. Type II cyst, which involves the lateral wall of the common bile duct, is also called an extra-hepatic supraduodenal biliary diverticulum. Type III cyst choledochal is a cystic dilatation of the duodenal intramural segment of the common bile duct. It can also have a mass effect while protruding into the lumen of the duodenum. Todani identified type IV cyst also as multiple extrahepatic biliary cysts. It could be either isolated in extrahepatic bile duct (type IVb) or combined with multiple large intrahepatic biliary cysts (type IVa). Type V cyst, on the other hand, is known as Caroli disease. It is characterized by multiple large and small intrahepatic biliary dilatations. Coexistence of Caroli disease and congenital hepatic fibrosis is called Caroli syndrome. In 2004, Visser proposed a revised classification to facilitate the diagnosis and management of choledochal bile duct malformations [53]. Here, the spectrum of Todani type I and type IV anomalies was classified under the name of congenital choledochal cyst. Type II koledokal divertikül and type III koledokosel. Likewise, depending on the way it manifests, Caroli disease or syndrome was called type V. In the Visser's classification, congenital choledochal cysts (Todani types I and IV) consist of focal or diffuse extrahepatic bile duct dilatation with varying degrees of intrahepatic involvement. It is the most common type of malformation with incidence rates of approximately 1/100,000–1/150,000. Common duct syndrome is the most commonly considered cause. Other proposed causes include increased intraluminal pressure due to narrow biliary stricture (stenosis), abnormal recanalization during organogenesis, reovirus infection, and insufficient ganglion cells in narrow bile duct part resulting in dilatation [8, 38].

4. Choledochal diverticulum

A choledochal diverticulum (Todani type II) is described as outpouching in the extrahepatic supraduodenal common bile duct. It is rare, has an incidence rate of less than 1/1,000,000 and accounts for approximately 2% of Todani-type malformations [2, 6]. It is a true diverticulum lined with biliary epithelium [2]. Histologically, it is similar to gallbladder duplication. It is associated with the common bile duct with a thin stalk. Increased intraluminal pressure as a result of sphincter of Oddi dysfunction was suggested as the cause.

5. Choledocele

It was first described by Courcy Wheeler in 1940 [54]. Choledochoceles (Todani type III) are poorly understood entities of the choledochal malformations. It is different from other choledochal cysts (CCs). True choledochoceles are the dilated segment of the common bile duct that prolapses or herniates into the small intestine [2, 55]. Their origin has long been the subject of debate. One hypothesis is that these cysts may be caused by an anomaly acquired by the ampulla of Vater's rudimentary lower embryonic bud or by dysfunction or obstruction of the sphincter of Oddi [56]. Although multiple etiological factors are considered, the most commonly blamed factor is inflammation after stone (calculus) passage or damage to the wall. It could be lined with biliary epithelium or ectopic mucosa of the intestine, or it may lie completely bare. It is very rare with an incidence rate of less than 1/1,000,000. It accounts for 1–4% of choledochal malformations [6]. Its differential diagnosis from submucosal duodenal lesions or periampullary duodenal duplication cysts is difficult. The diagnosis is typically made by cholangiography or endoscopic ultrasonography [57].

6. Caroli disease and syndrome

It was first defined by French gastroenterologists in 1958 as congenital multiple intrahepatic cystic dilatation pattern. Caroli disease (Todani type V) is a rare autosomal recessive disorder. It is the second most common type of malformation. It is observed at a ratio of 6–30% in the West and 18–19% in the East. It is the most common type of choledochal malformation with an incidence rate of approximately 1/500,000 in Western countries [2, 6]. Caroli disease is characterized by *in utero* malformation product of the ductal plate and congenital intrahepatic ectasia of the bile duct. When Caroli disease is observed together with congenital hepatic fibrosis, it is called Caroli syndrome [2, 6]. The intrahepatic biliary tract originates from monolayer cells around the portal branches, called the ductal plate [55]. These cell layers are structured to produce small ducts in the periphery and large bile ducts in the hilum.

Ductal plate malformation at the level of the great bile duct results in Caroli disease [2, 58]. Imaging studies show varying size of intrahepatic saccular cystic structures associated with the biliary system. On MRI and CT, it appears as ectatic bile ducts around enlarged portal branches. It is called the central dot sign, which is thought to be highly indicative for the diagnosis of Caroli disease [2]. Complications of Caroli disease include intraductal stone formation due to bile stasis and recurrent cholangitis [2, 6]. Besides causing intrahepatic cysts by blocking the large bile ducts, Caroli syndrome also affects peripheral bile ducts as a result of congenital hepatic fibrosis [2, 59]. Associated conditions include congenital choledochal cysts, cholangiocarcinoma (7–10% incidence), autosomal recessive polycystic kidney disease, and renal cystic diseases involving medullary sponge kidney [2]. Here, the association of renal and hepatic diseases is the common genetic locus (PKHD1 gene on 6p21 chromosomal region) [58].

7. Complications

Complications of common bile duct malformations range from cholestasis with stone formation to recurrent cholangitis, pancreatitis, biliary and hepatic fibrosis, and malignant transformation (cholangiocarcinoma). Cholestasis is the result of external compression of a large extrahepatic cystic malformation causing a regional mass effect or inadequate prolonged biliary drainage by the malformed biliary tract [60]. Stone formation can occur anywhere along the affected biliary system. Recurrent cholangitis and cholecystitis are probably multifactorial. The reasons blamed for this are static lithogenic bile salts as well as chronic inflammation, reflux of pancreatic enzymes, and intestinal bacterial reflux [2]. Regardless of the underlying cause, recurrent cholangitis attacks lead to fibrosis in the cyst wall, ductal sclerosis, and an increased risk of malignant degeneration [6]. Hepatic fibrosis may develop when chronic inflammation affects the intrahepatic biliary system as in congenital choledochal cysts (Todani type IVa) and Caroli disease (Todani type V). Malignant transformation is the best known and feared complication of choledochal malformations. The thesis that chronic inflammation in the malformation-affected biliary system results in cellular dysplasia is assumed to be correct. Chronic inflammation destroys protective mucin-producing epithelial cells. This effect is also enhanced by carcinogen products such as bile salts metabolized by *Escherichia coli*.

The risk of developing malignancy is between 6% and 30% in patients with choledochal cysts. This risk is low in childhood (<1%) but increases by 30–40% at the age of more than 50 years [45, 61]. The malignancy of choledochal cysts originates from both the gallbladder and the choledochal. In a large-scale Japanese study with patients who had choledochal cysts and developed cancer, 62.3% had gallbladder cancer, 32.1% bile duct cancer, and 4.7% had both, which was consistent with other reports [15, 62]. Gallbladder cancer is found in 5% of choledochal cyst patients with PBM [63]. An evaluation of the adult cohort revealed that this is usually observed in the sixth or seventh decade of life [64]. With the cumulative effect of biliary stasis and chronic inflammation itself, the risk of malignancy increases with age [2, 7]. Cholangiocarcinoma develops in a small subgroup of patients (0.7–3%), especially in type I and IV, after surgical resection [18, 22, 65, 66]. This shows that the risk of malignancy does not completely regress after resection in this group of patients. The etiology of this residual malignancy is unclear. Many studies performed in the East and West do not have follow-up periods long enough to determine persistent risk because it takes more than three decades to occur [67, 68]. However, currently, there is a 6% risk of malignancy after complete cyst resection, while there is a 33% risk of malignancy after incomplete cyst resection [69]. The most common type of cancer is adenocarcinoma, followed by anaplastic carcinoma, undifferentiated carcinoma, and squamous cell carcinoma [70]. About 70% of malignancies originate from the cystic wall. Cholangiocarcinoma in adults and rhabdomyocarcinoma or adenocarcinoma in children are frequently observed. Twenty-four percent of them originate from the gallbladder. The remaining 6% are hepatocellular carcinoma and pancreatic carcinoma [7, 70, 71]. Intrahepatic cysts have a low malignant potential depending on the extent of the involved area and the extent of inflammation and hepatic parenchymal atrophy [20, 72, 73]. Among the different types of choledochal malformations, extrahepatic choledochal cysts (Todani types I and IV) have the highest risk of developing cancer. They are followed by intrahepatic choledochal cysts (Todani type IVa), Caroli disease (Todani type V), choledochal diverticulum (Todani type II), and choledochocele (Todani type III). A surveillance strategy is proposed for patients treated primarily for cyst types I and IV and unresected type V using annual liver function tests, Ca 19–9 measurement and biannual ultrasound assessment for 20 years post cyst resection, with biannual liver function testing, Ca 19–9 measurement and 3-yearly ultrasound assessment thereafter [74]. it has been opined that long- term follow-up strategies might not be associated with a better prognosis. One report suggested that follow-up with regular clinic reviews alone does not affect the resectability of cholangiocarcinoma [75].

8. Surgical treatment

Surgical treatment should be based on the extent of biliary involvement based on the widely used Todani classification and anatomical findings and the presence or absence of PBM [76]. The treatment goal for choledochal malformations is to eliminate the risk of malignancy and to treat complications. Surgical treatment depends on the localization and size of the cyst rather than the morphological features [53, 55, 72]. The standard treatment in most CCs is the resection of the bile duct up to the lobar bifurcation, specifically toward the pancreatic parenchyma close to the pancreatic duct junction. Biliary tract continuity is provided by roux-en-Y hepaticojejunostomy (HJ), hepaticoduodenostomy (HD), or jejunal interposition [64, 77, 78]. Hepaticoduodenostomy presents an effective approach to biliary reconstruction following surgical interventions for choledochal cysts. It presents a faster alternative to hepa ticojejunostomy in both operative times and length of stay, with similar rates of complications, including the feared cholangitis [79]. Proximal cyst excision is a non-precisely programmable procedure that needs attention to preserve the portal vein and hepatic artery. Although extrahepatic congenital choledochal cysts usually require complete excision of the entire extrahepatic biliary tree using cholecystectomy and hepaticojejunostomy, more conservative surgical options can be used if there is limited involvement in the distal bile duct, and the interventional approach is based on a 3-cm-size threshold [5, 60]. When the cyst extends into the pancreas, its management is critical and sometimes challenging. During recurrent cholangitis attacks, adhesions in the tissues surrounding the portal vein and pancreas could develop. For these reasons, complete excision may not be possible due to peritoneal infection, bleeding, and the risk of postoperative pancreatic leak [80–82]. The residual intrapancreatic portion of the choledochal cyst hosts multiple pathological changes such as pancreatitis, secondary calculus in the bile duct, and even carcinogenesis [83, 84]. Acute pancreatitis is often secondary to the intrapancreatic portion of the postoperative residual choledochal cyst [85]. Residual postoperative intrapancreatic choledochal cyst may also lead to secondary carcinogenesis and associated morbidity. Some previous reports showed that stone formation not only stimulates cancer, but also some carcinogenic factors may exist in the residual intrapancreatic part of the choledochal cyst [86]. These findings indicated the necessity of surgical excision of asymptomatic residual choledochal cysts. Intrapancreatic choledochal cysts carry a 0.7–6.0% risk of malignant transformation [5]. There has been no consensus so far on whether excision of the intrapancreatic common bile duct cyst is necessary if there are no clinical symptoms. At the same time, the optimal timing of surgery is unclear. The proximal and distal endpoint of the biliary malformation including involvement of the ampulla of Vater expanding into the pancreatic head should be determined preoperatively [72]. Generally, the localization of the pancreatic cyst is inside the head of the pancreas, close to the neck and to the left of the bile duct [87]. Investigation and differentiation of a residual intrapancreatic choledochal cyst should be started from the back and right side of the pancreatic head. Then, it is gradually deepened into the left field. During this procedure, the direction of the bile duct is confirmed at intervals by fine needle aspiration and finger control [88]. The separation should be close to the bile duct wall. When the lumen terminates abruptly near the end of the bile duct, attention should be paid to the junction of the pancreatic and bile ducts. The diagnosis of a residual intrapancreatic cyst is relatively easy with type-B ultrasonography, CT, and magnetic resonance cholangiopancreatography (MRCP) [89]. Preoperative MRCP examination is crucial to prevent pancreatic duct injury during surgery. It clearly shows the specific anatomy of the pancreatobiliary junction [90]. Different cholangiopancreatography angles of duct reveal the angle of the cholangio-pancreatic duct junction, the rough flow direction to the main pancreatic duct, and the length of the stenosed portion of the lower portion of the bile duct [91].

Because of the high risk of malignancy arising from inadequate resection of the mucosa, any residual area should be excised and always followed up regularly. It is difficult to distinguish pathological changes in choledochal cysts from the inflammatory bile duct. The extent of the excision is mainly based on radiological and intraoperative findings. Surgical treatment is ideally adopted for type I CC. In Todani type IV with intrahepatic and extrahepatic cysts, extrahepatic cysts should be definitively excised. If intrahepatic cysts are limited, biliary-enteric reconstruction is performed along with partial hepatectomy. Especially in patients with bilobar involvement and with diffuse intrahepatic dilatation associated with complications such as stones, cholangitis, and biliary cirrhosis, liver transplantation should be considered [92, 93]. In the distal management of choledochal cysts, if there is no relationship between the choledochal cyst and the pancreatic duct in the preoperative imaging, the distal cyst is excised at a distance of about 5 mm at the junction with the pancreatic duct of the visible bile duct, and the stump is sutured [94]. If the choledochal cyst extends to the junction of the pancreatic duct, the same procedure is adopted. Sometimes, the insufficiency of the ampulla of Vater is observed along with a cylindrical cyst. The distal end of the choledochal cyst opens directly into the duodenum with the insufficient ampulla, and the pancreatic duct appears to be attached to the cyst. In this case, the cylindrical cyst and papilla are excised, and duodenum mucosa and pancreatic duct are subjected to ductoplasty as a modified procedure of local excision of early noninvasive adenocarcinoma and benign lesions in the papilla. Secondary infections may require antibiotics, drainage, and sometimes surgery. Partial hepatectomy and liver transplantation are disputable. However, it is successful in the presence of diffuse intrahepatic ductal dilatation, stenosis, and multiple intraluminal stones [72]. If resection is not performed, long-term follow-up of intrahepatic biliary cysts is required [20, 72]. Despite their low malignant potential, choledochal diverticula (Todani type II) are prophylactically excised to prevent the sequelae of compression effect on adjacent structures [55]. Usually, these cysts are ligated at the neck and excised without the need for reconstruction of bile duct [12]. However, sometimes extrahepatic bile duct excision may be required. In this case, sometimes patients with tight adhesion of the diverticulum to the extra- or intrahepatic biliary tract due to inflammation may be encountered. Releasing the diverticulum from the bile duct could be technically challenging [95]. The isolated segment is removed, and primary repair is performed via T-tube with a low recurrence rate without the need for cholecystectomy [60, 96]. Choledochoceles, which are very similar to choledochal diverticulum, have a low malignant potential of approximately 2.5% throughout life [5]. If they cause biliary or intestinal obstruction, they are excised [6, 55, 56]. Due to the low risk of malignancy, unroofing (endoscopic or transduodenal sphincteroplasty) or transduodenal excision (in large cysts) is the optimal treatment. Endoscopic monitoring should be considered for younger patients treated with sphincterotomy. The prognosis of Caroli disease or syndrome depends on the extent of involvement, but is generally poor. Localized disease is treated with prophylactic hepatic lobectomy. Recurrent and life-threatening cholangitis, liver failure, cirrhosis, portal hypertension, or malignant disease requires orthotopic liver transplantation [97, 98]. Surgical treatment options include laparoscopic treatment. Its main advantages include excellent visualization and low blood loss [99]. In addition, it has better postoperative recovery, less surgical trauma and postoperative pain, less abdominal wall trauma, less cavity drainage time, reduced postoperative paralytic ileus time, and shorter hospital stay. The overall complication and mortality rates are also lower compared with the series involving treatment with open surgery [100, 101]. Recent report supports HD as an effective alternative to the conventional Roux-en-Y HJ reconstruction in laparoscopic excision of choledochal cyst in children [102]. Exposure of the anastomotic site and IHBD is very difficult to achieve by conventional endoscopy. DBE provides a direct view of these sites and enables diagnostic assessment and minimally invasive therapy to be performed simultaneously. It will replace more invasive treatments such as percutaneous transhepatic intervention and surgical procedures [103].

Author details

Umut Tüysüz
Department of Liver Transplantation Surgery, Hamidiye Etfal Education and Research Hospital, Istanbul, Turkey

*Address all correspondence to: umutuysuz@gmail.com

References

[1] Liu Y, Yao X, Li S, et al. Comparison of therapeutic effects of laparoscopic and open operation for congenital choledochal cysts in adults. Gastroenterology Research and Practice. 2014;**2014**:670260

[2] Singham J, Yoshida EM, Scudamore CH. Choledochal cysts. Part 1. Classification and pathogenesis. Canadian Journal of Surgery. 2009;**52**:434-440

[3] Liu CL, Fan ST, Lo CM, et al. Choledochal cysts in adults. Archives of Surgery. 2002;**137**:465-468

[4] Levy AD, Rohrmann CA. Biliary cystic disease. Current Problems in Diagnostic Radiology. 2003;**32**:233-263

[5] Singham J, Yoshida EM, Scudamore CH. Choledochal cysts. Part 3. Management. Canadian Journal of Surgery. 2010;**53**:51-56

[6] Soares KC, Arnaoutakis DJ, Kamel I, et al. Choledochal cysts: Presentation, clinical differentiation, and management. Journal of the American College of Surgeons. 2014;**219**: 1167-1180

[7] Sastry AV, Abbadessa B, Wayne MG, Steele JG, Cooperman AM. What is the incidence of biliary carcinoma in choledochal cysts, when do they develop, and how should it affect management? World Journal of Surgery. 2015;**39**:487-492

[8] Katabathina VS, Kapalczynski W, Dasyam AK, Anaya-Baez V, Menias CO. Adult choledochal cysts: Current update on classification, pathogenesis, and cross-sectional imaging findings. Abdominal Imaging. 2015;**40**:1971-1981

[9] Kimura K, Ohto M, Ono T, Tsuchiya Y, Saisho H, Kawamura K, et al. Congenital cystic dilatation of the common bile duct: Relationship to anomalous pancreaticobiliary ductal union. AJR. American Journal of Roentgenology. 1977;**128**(4):571-577

[10] Funabiki T, Matsubara T, MiyakawaS, IshiharaS. Pancreaticobiliary maljunction and carcinogenesis to biliary and pancreatic malignancy. Langenbeck's Archives of Surgery. 2009;**394**:159-169

[11] Nicholl M, Pitt HA, Wolf P, Cooney J, Kalayoglu M, Shilyansky J, et al. Choledochal cysts in western adults: Complexities compared to children. Journal of Gastrointestinal Surgery. 2004;**8**:245-252

[12] Babbitt DP. Congenital choledochal cysts: New etiological concept based on anomalous relationships of the common bile duct and pancreatic bulb. Annales de Radiologie (Paris). 1969;**12**:231-240

[13] García Cano J, Godoy MA, Morillas Ariño J, Pérez García JI. Pancreatobiliary maljunction. Not only an eastern disease. Anales de Medicina Interna. 2007;**24**:384-386

[14] Kamisawa T, Honda G, Kurata M, Tokura M, Tsuruta K. Pancreatobiliary disorders associated with pancreaticobiliary maljunction. Digestive Surgery. 2010;**27**:100-104

[15] Bhavsar MS, Vora HB, Giriyappa VH. Choledochal cysts: A review of literature. Saudi Journal of Gastroenterology. 2012;**18**:230-236

[16] Lipsett PA, Pitt HA, Colombani PM, et al. Choledochal cyst disease. A

changing pattern of presentation. Annals of Surgery. 1994;**220**:644-652

[17] Shi LB, Peng SY, Meng XK, Peng CH, Liu YB, Chen XP, et al. Diagnosis and treatment of congenital choledochal cyst: 20 years' experience in China. World Journal of Gastroenterology. 2001;**7**:732-734

[18] Soares KC, Kim Y, Spolverato G, Maithel S, Bauer TW, Marques H, et al. Presentation and clinical outcomes of Choledochal cysts in children and adults: A multi-institutional analysis. JAMA Surgery. 2015;**150**:577-584

[19] Kinoshita H, Nagata E, Hirohashi K, Sakai K, Kobayashi Y. Carcinoma of the gallbladder with an anomalous connection between the choledochus and the pancreatic duct. Report of 10 cases and review of the literature in Japan. Cancer. 1984;**54**:762-769

[20] He XD, Wang L, Liu W, Liu Q, Qu Q, Li BL, et al. The risk of carcinogenesis in congenital choledochal cyst patients: An analysis of 214 cases. Annals of Hepatology. 2014;**13**:819-826

[21] Baumann R, Uettwiller H, Duclos B, Jouin H, Kerschen A, Adloff M, et al. Congenital cystic dilatation of the common bile duct, anomaly of the biliopancreatic junction and cancer of the bile ducts. Gastroentérologie Clinique et Biologique. 1987;**11**(12):849-855

[22] Lee SE, Jang JY, Lee YJ, et al. Choledochal cyst and associated malignant tumors in adults: A multicenter survey in South Korea. Archives of Surgery. 2011;**146**(10):1178-1184

[23] Tashiro S, Imaizumi T, Ohkawa H, Okada A, Katoh T, Kawaharada Y, et al. Pancreaticobiliary maljunction: Retrospective and nationwide survey in Japan. Journal of Hepato-Biliary-Pancreatic Surgery. 2003;**10**(5):345-351

[24] Kamisawa T, Ando H, Suyama M, Shimada M, Morine Y, Shi-Mada H, et al. Japanese clinical practice guidelines for pancreaticobiliary maljunction. Journal of Gastroenterology. 2012;**7**(7):731-759

[25] Komi N, Udaka H, Ikeda N, Kashiwagi Y. Congenital dilatation of the biliary tract; new classification and study with particular reference to anomalous arrangement of the pancreaticobiliary ducts. Gastroenterologia Japonica. 1977;**12**(4):293-304

[26] Okada A, Hasegawa T, Oguchi Y, Nakamura T. Recent advances in pathophysiology and surgical treatment of congenital dilatation of the bile duct. Journal of Hepato-Biliary-Pancreatic Surgery. 2002;**9**:342-351

[27] Imazu M, Iwai N, Tokiwa K, Shimotake T, Kimura O, Ono S. Factors of biliary carcinogenesis in choledochal cysts. European Journal of Pediatric Surgery. 2001;**11**:24-27

[28] Mabrut JY, Kianmanesh R, Nuzzo G, Castaing D, Boudjema K, Le'toublon C, et al. Surgical management of congenital intrahepatic bile duct dilatation, Caroli's disease and syndrome: Long-term results of the French Association of Surgery Multicenter study. Annals of Surgery. 2013;**258**(5):713-721

[29] Okada A. Forme fruste choledochal cyst. Journal of Pediatric Surgery. 1986;**21**(4):383

[30] Shimotakahara A, Yamataka A, Kobayashi H, Okada Y, Yanai T, Lane GJ, et al. Forme fruste choledochal cyst: Long-term follow-up with special reference to surgical technique. Journal of Pediatric Surgery. 2003;**38**(12):1833-1836

[31] Kamisawa T, Anjiki H, Egawa N, Kurata M, Honda G, Tsuruta K. Diagnosis and clinical implications of pancreatobiliary reflux. World Journal of Gastroenterology. 2008;**14**(43):6622-6626

[32] Misra SP, Dwivedi M. Pancreaticobiliary ductal union. Gut. 1990;**31**(10):1144-1149

[33] Todani T, Watanabe Y, Narusue M, Tabuchi K, Okajima K. Congenital bile duct cysts: Classification, operative procedures, and review of thirty-seven cases including cancer arising from choledochal cyst. American Journal of Surgery. 1977;**134**(2):263-269

[34] Todani T, Watanabe Y, Toki A, et al. Carcinoma related to choledochal cysts with internal drainage operations. Surgery, Gynecology and Obstetrics. 1987;**164**:61-64

[35] Flanigan DP. Biliary carcinoma associated with biliary cysts. Cancer. 1977;**40**:880-883

[36] Soares KC, Goldstein SD, Ghaseb MA, Kamel I, Hackam DJ, Pawlik TM. Pediatric choledochal cysts: Diagnosis and current management. Pediatric Surgery International. 2017;**33**:637-650

[37] Rozel C, Garel L, Rypens F, et al. Imaging of biliary disorders in children. Pediatric Radiology. 2011;**41**:208-220

[38] Lewis VA, Adam SZ, Nikolaidis P, et al. Imaging of choledochal cysts. Abdominal Imaging. 2015;**40**:1567-1580

[39] Park DH, Kim MH, Lee SK, Lee SS, Choi JS, Lee YS, et al. Can MRCP replace the diagnostic role of ERCP for patients with choledochal cysts? Gastrointestinal Endoscopy. 2005;**62**:360-366

[40] Park KB, Auh YH, Kim JH, et al. Diagnostic pit falls in the cholangiographic diagnosis of choledochoceles: Cholangiographic quality and its effect on visualization. Abdominal Imaging. 2001;**26**:48-54

[41] Irie H, Honda H, Jimi M, Yokohata K, Chijiiwa K, Kuroiwa T, et al. Value of MR cholangiopancreatography in evaluating choledochal cysts. AJR. American Journal of Roentgenology. 1998;**171**:1381-1385

[42] Huang CT, Lee HC, Chen WT, Jiang CB, Shih SL, Yeung CY. Usefulness of magnetic resonance cholangiopancreatography in pancreatobiliary abnormalities in pediatric patients. Pediatrics and Neonatology. 2011;**52**(6):332-336

[43] Han BK, Babcock DS, Gelfand MH. Choledochal cyst with bile duct dilatation: Sonography and 99mTc IDA cholescintigraphy. AJR. 1981;**136**:1075-1079

[44] Saito T, Terui K, Mitsunaga T, Nakata M, Yoshida H. Significance of imaging modalities for preoperative evaluation of the pancreaticobiliary system in surgery for pediatric choledochal cyst. Journal of Hepato-Biliary-Pancreatic Sciences. 2016;**23**:347-352

[45] Edil BH, Cameron JL, Reddy S, Lum Y, Lipsett PA, Nathan H, et al. Choledochal cyst disease in children and adults: A 30-year single-institution experience. Journal of the American College of Surgeons. 2008;**206**:1000-1005; discussion 1005-8

[46] Gupta N, Gupta V, Noushif M, et al. Unusual presentations of choledochal cyst: Case series and review of literature. The Indian Journal of Surgery. 2015;**77**:1318-1322

[47] Forny DN, Ferrante SM, Silveira VG, Siviero I, Chagas VL, Méio IB. Choledochal cyst in childhood: Review of 30 cases. Revista do Colégio Brasileiro de Cirurgiões. 2014;**41**(5):331-335

[48] Subramony R, Kittisarapong N, Barata I, Nelson M. Choledochal cyst mimicking gallbladder with stones in a six-year-old with right-sided abdominal pain. The Western Journal of Emergency Medicine. 2015;**16**(4):568-571

[49] Shindo K, Aishima S, Ohuchida K, et al. Podoplanin expression in the cyst wall correlates with the progression of intraductal papillary mucinous neoplasm. Virchows Archiv. 2014;**465**:265-273

[50] Gadelhak N, Shehta A, Hamed H. Diagnosis and management of choledochal cyst: 20 years of single center experience. World Journal of Gastroenterology. 2014;**20**:7061-7066

[51] Chen W, Liu Q, Tan SY, et al. Association between carcinoembryonic antigen, carbohydrate antigen 19-9 and body mass index in colorectal cancer patients. Molecular and Clinical Oncology. 2013;**1**:879-886

[52] Alonso-Lej F, Rever WB, Pessagno DJ. Congenital choledochal cyst, with a report of 2, and an analysis of 94, cases. International Abstracts of Surgery. 1959;**108**:1-30

[53] Visser BC, Suh I, Way LW, Kang SM. Congenital choledochal cysts in adults. Archives of Surgery. 1960;**2004**(139):855-860; discussion, 860-862

[54] de Courcy Wheeler WI. An unusual case of obstruction to the common bile-duct (choledochocele?). BJS. 1940;**27**:446-448

[55] Martin RF. Biliary cysts: A review and simplified classification scheme. The Surgical Clinics of North America. 2015;**94**:219-232

[56] Law R, Topazian M. Diagnosis and treatment of choledochoceles. Clinical Gastroenterology and Hepatology. 2014;**12**:196-203

[57] Scholz FJ, Carrera GF, Larsen CR. The choledochocele: Correlation of radiological, clinical and pathological findings. Radiology. 1976;**118**:25-28

[58] Sato Y, Ren XS, Nakanuma Y. Caroli's disease: Current knowledge of its biliary pathogenesis obtained from an orthologous rat model. Internaticonal Journal of Hepatology. 2012;**2012**:1-10

[59] Bismuth H, Krissat J. Choledochal cystic malignancies. Annals of Oncology. 1999;**10**(suppl 4):94-98

[60] Lipsett PA, Pitt HA. Surgical treatment of choledochal cysts. Journal of Hepato-Biliary-Pancreatic Surgery. 2003;**10**:352-359

[61] Søreide K, Søreide JA. Bile duct cyst as precursor to biliary tract cancer. Annals of Surgical Oncology. 2007;**14**:1200-1211

[62] Mori H, Iida H, Maehira H, Kitamura N, Shimizu T, Tani M. Synchronous primary gallbladder and pancreatic cancer associated with congenital biliary dilatation and pancreaticobiliary maljunction. Surgical Case Reports. 2017;**3**:113

[63] Chijiiwa K, Kimura H, Tanaka M. Malignant potential of the gallbladder in patients with anomalous pancreaticobiliary ductal junction. The difference in risk between patients with and without choledochal cyst. International Surgery. 1995;**80**:61-64

[64] Ishibashi H, Shimada M, Kamisawa T, Fujii H, Hamada Y, Kubota M, et al. Japanese clinical practice guidelines for congenital biliary dilatation. Journal of Hepato-Biliary-Pancreatic Sciences. 2017;**24**:1-16

[65] Watanabe Y, Toki A, Todani T. Bile duct cancer developed after cyst excision for choledochal cyst. Journal of Hepato-Biliary-Pancreatic Surgery. 1999;**6**:207-212

[66] Ng WT. Bile duct carcinogenesis after excision of extrahepatic bile ducts in pancreaticobiliary maljunction. Surgery. 2000;**128**:492-494

[67] Takeshita N, Ota T, Yamamoto M. Forty-year experience with flow-diversion surgery for patients with congenital choledochal cysts with pancreaticobiliary maljunction at a single institution. Annals of Surgery. 2011;**254**:1050-1053

[68] Kobayashi S, Asano T, Yamasaki M, Kenmochi T, Nakagohri T, Ochiai T. Risk of bile duct carcinogenesis after excision of extrahepatic bile ducts in pancreaticobiliary maljunction. Surgery. 1999;**126**:939-944

[69] Liu YB, Wang JW, Devkota KR, Ji ZL, Li JT, Wang XA, et al. Congenital choledochal cysts in adults: Twenty-five-year experience. Chinese Medical Journal. 2007;**120**:1404-1407

[70] Fieber SS, Nance FC. Choledochal cyst and neoplasm: A comprehensive review of 106 cases and presentation of two original cases. The American Surgeon. 1997;**63**:982-987

[71] Todani T, Tabuchi K, Watanabe Y, Kobayashi T. Carcinoma arising in the wall of congenital bile duct cysts. Cancer. 1979;**44**:1134-1141

[72] Ronnekleiv-Kelly SM, Soares KC, Ejaz A, Pawlik TM. Management of choledochal cysts. Current Opinion in Gastroenterology. 2016;**32**:225-231

[73] Ohashi T, Wakai T, Kubota M, et al. Risk of subsequent biliary malignancy in patients undergoing cyst excision for congenital choledochal cysts: Biliary malignancy after cyst excision. Journal of Gastroenterology and Hepatology. 2013;**28**:243-247

[74] Koea J, O'Grady M, Agraval J, Srinivasa S. Defining an optimal surveillance strategy for patients following choledochal cyst resection: Results of a systematic review. ANZ Journal of Surgery. 2022;**92**(6):1356-1364

[75] Ng DW, Chiow AK, Poh WT, Tan SS. Metachronous cholangiocarcinoma 13 years post resection of choledochal cyst-is long-term follow-up useful?: A case study and review of the literature. Surgical Case Reports. 2016;**2**:60

[76] Le RB, Gagnière J, Filaire L, et al. Pancreaticobiliary maljunction and choledochal cysts: From embryogenesis to therapeutics aspects. Surgical and Radiologic Anatomy. 2016;**38**:1053-1060

[77] Moslim MA, Takahashi H, Seifarth FG, Walsh RM, Morris-Stiff G. Choledochal cyst disease in a Western center: A 30-year experience. Journal of Gastrointestinal Surgery. 2016;**20**:1453-1463

[78] Kim Y, Hyun JJ, Lee JM, Lee HS, Kim CD. Anomalous union of the pancreaticobiliary duct without choledochal cyst: Is cholecystectomy alone sufficient? Langenbeck's Archives of Surgery. 2014;**399**:1071-1076

[79] Gonzalez DEH, Medrano AR, De Leon SUV. Biliary reconstruction after choledochal cyst resection: A systematic review and meta-analysis on hepaticojejunostomy

vs hepaticoduodenostomy. Pediatric Surgery International. 2021;**37**(10):1313-1322

[80] Saluja SS, Nayeem M, Sharma BC, et al. Management of choledochal cysts and their complications. The American Surgeon. 2012;**78**:284-290

[81] Jordan PH, Goss JA, Rosenberg WR, et al. Some considerations for management of choledochal cysts. American Journal of Surgery. 2004;**187**:790-795

[82] Cho MJ, Hwang S, Lee YJ, et al. Surgical experience of 204 cases of adult choledochal cyst disease over 14 years. World Journal of Surgery. 2011;**35**:1094-1102

[83] Wang WJ, Lv ZD, Yang ZC, et al. Prrx1 enhanced the migration ability of breast cancer cell by initiating epithelial-mesenchymal transition. Cancer Cell Research. 2017;**4**:362-367

[84] Chen TT, Liu YQ, Lin BD, et al. Effects of RNA interference of the eno1 gene on the malignant biological behaviors of gastric cell lines. Cancer Cell Research. 2017;**4**:326-333

[85] Ando H, Kaneko K, Ito T, et al. Complete excision of the intrapancreatic portion of choledochal cysts. Journal of the American College of Surgeons. 1996;**183**:317-321

[86] Fan F et al. Clinical significance of intrapancreatic choledochal cyst excision in surgical management of type I choledochal cyst. The Journal of International Medical Research. Mar 2018;**46**(3):1221-1229

[87] Ryu M, Takayama W, Watanabe K, et al. Ventral pancreatic resection for adenoma and low-grade malignancies of the head of the pancreas. Surgery Today. 1996;**26**:476-481

[88] Kolb A, Kleeff J, Frohlich B, et al. Resection of the intrapancreatic bile duct preserving the pancreas. Journal of Hepato-Biliary-Pancreatic Surgery. 2009;**16**:31-34

[89] Shimizu T, Suzuki R, Yamashiro Y, et al. Magnetic resonance cholangiopancreatography in assessing the cause of acute pancreatitis in children. Pancreas. 2001;**22**:196-199

[90] Yoon JH. Magnetic resonance cholangiopancreatography diagnosis of choledochal cyst involving the cystic duct: Report of three cases. The British Journal of Radiology. 2011;**84**:e18-e22

[91] Jara H, Barish MA, Yucel EK, et al. MR hydrography: Theory and practice of static fluid imaging. AJR. American Journal of Roentgenology. 1998;**170**:873-882

[92] Xia HT, Dong JH, Yang T, Zeng JP, Liang B. Extrahepatic cyst excision and partial hepatectomy for Todani type IV-A cysts. Digestive and Liver Disease. 2014;**46**:1025-1030

[93] Cerwenka H. Bile duct cyst in adults: Interventional treatment, resection, or transplantation? World Journal of Gastroenterology. 2013;**19**:5207-5211

[94] Xia HT, Yang T, Liang B, et al. Treatment and outcomes of adults with remnant intrapancreatic choledochal cysts. Surgery. 2016;**159**:418-425

[95] Ouaïssi M, Kianmanesh R, Belghiti J, Ragot E, Mentha G, Adham M, et al. Gigot JF; working Group of the French Surgical Association. Todani type II congenital bile duct cyst: European multicenter study of the French surgical association and literature review. Annals of Surgery. 2015;**262**:130-138

[96] Wiseman K, Buczkowski AK, Chung SW, FrancoEur J, Schaeffer D,

Scudamore CH. Epidemiology, presentation, diagnosis, and outcomes of choledochal cysts in adults in an urban environment. American Journal of Surgery. 2005;**189**:527-531; discussion, 531

[97] Bockhorn M, Malagó M, Lang H, et al. The role of surgery in Caroli's disease. Journal of the American College of Surgeons. 2006;**202**:928-932

[98] Habib S, Shakil O, Couto OF, et al. Caroli's disease and orthotopic liver transplantation. Liver Transplantation. 2006;**12**:416-421

[99] Liuming H, Hongwu Z, Gang L, Jun J, Wenying H, Wong KK, et al. The effect of laparoscopic excision vs open excision in children with choledochal cyst: A midterm follow-up study. Journal of Pediatric Surgery. 2011;**46**(4):662-665

[100] Liem NT, Pham HD, Vu HM. Is the laparoscopic operation as safe as open operation for choledochal cyst in children? Journal of Laparoendoscopic & Advanced Surgical Techniques. Part A. 2011;**21**(4):367-370

[101] Wang B, Feng Q, Mao JX, Liu L, Wong KK. Early experience with laparoscopic excision of choledochal cyst in 41 children. Journal of Pediatric Surgery. 2012;**47**(12):2175-2178

[102] Yeung F, Fung ACH, Chung PHY, Wong KKY. Short-term and long-term outcomes after roux- en-Y hepaticojejunostomy versus hepaticoduodenostomy following laparoscopic excision of choledochal cyst in children. Surgical Endoscopy. May 2020;**34**(5):2172-2177

[103] Mukai M, Kaji T, Masuya R. Long-term outcomes of surgery for choledochal cysts: A single-institution study focusing on follow-up and late complications. Surgery Today. 2018;**48**(9):835-840

Section 4

Gallbladder Cancer

Chapter 5

Gallbladder Cancer: Diagnosis and Surgical Management

Asmita Chopra and Alessandro Paniccia

Abstract

Gallbladder cancer (GBCa) is a biliary tract malignancy that is common in South America and Southeast Asia, where patients often present with abdominal pain and jaundice. However, most cases of GBCa in the United States are diagnosed incidentally following cholecystectomy. The pre-operative diagnosis and evaluation involves imaging with ultrasound, CT, MRI, and PET. In patients with incidental GBCa, the histopathology directs further management. The surgical management of GBCa ranges from a simple cholecystectomy to liver resection with lymphadenectomy. Bile duct and vascular resections are reserved to obtain negative margins. To date, multiple controversies remain in the management of GBCa. The determination of type of surgery is based predominantly on T stage. The need for liver resection for tumor on the peritonealized surface continues to be debated. The added value of neoadjuvant and peri-operative therapy is being actively investigated. Systemic therapy has greatly evolved encompassing the use of capecitabine, gemcitabine-cisplatin, with recent addition of taxanes, HER2 inhibitors, and immunotherapy using PD-L1 inhibitors including Durvalumab. This chapter describes current diagnosis and treatment practices for GBCa especially determinants of surgical management and the benefits of peri-operative systemic therapy highlighting the recent advances and shortcomings.

Keywords: gallbladder cancer, radical cholecystectomy, incidental cancer, neoadjuvant, PD-L1 inhibitors

1. Introduction

Gallbladder cancer (GBCa) is the most common form of biliary tract cancer and is associated with a particularly insidious course coupled with an aggressive biological behavior. While GBCa constitutes 40% of diagnosed biliary tract malignancies, the incidence has been reported to be as high as 80–95% in autopsy studies [1, 2]. Gallbladder cancer has the worst prognosis of all bile duct malignancies with a 5-year relative survival of 19% [1]. While rare in the developed world, including the United States, incidence of GBCa is high in South America and Southeast Asia, and is highest in women of North India [3]. The most important risk factor of GBCa is chronic cholelithiasis, with more than 85% cases of gallbladder cancer being associated with gallstones. Conversely, less than 3% of patients with gallstones, eventually develop gallbladder cancer. As such, there is no role for prophylactic cholecystectomy in patients with asymptomatic gallstone disease in the absence of high risk features such as associated polyps measuring more than 10 mm, and gallbladder wall thickening [4]. Females are two times more likely to develop GBCa compared to their male counterparts [5]. Additional risk factors of gallbladder cancer include: chronic inflammation, porcelain gallbladder, infections including bacterial (most commonly Salmonella and Helicobacter) and parasitic (Clonorchis and Opisthorchis), primary sclerosing cholangitis, smoking, obesity, gallbladder polyps, and family history of gallbladder cancer [4]. Additionally genetic mutations associated with other gastrointestinal malignancies—including TP53 mutation (47.1–59%), ERBB2/3 amplification (9.8–19%), CDKN2A/B loss (5.9–19%), ARID1A mutation (13%), KRAS mutation (4–13%), PIK3CA mutation (5.9–12.5%), NRAS mutation (6.3%) and BRAF mutation (1–5.9%)—have also been reported in GBCa [6]. In this chapter, we discuss the diagnosis of GBCa in patients with clinical symptoms as well as asymptomatic patients who are incidentally diagnosed on imaging or following pathological evaluation of a cholecystectomy specimen. We also discuss the various determinants of surgical and medical management of patients with GBCa, as well as the recent advances in treatment strategies.

2. Diagnosis of gallbladder cancer

2.1 Clinical presentation

Patients with gallbladder cancer may present with constitutive symptoms of weight loss and anorexia, and in advanced cases with abdominal pain, abdominal mass and jaundice. These symptoms are more commonly reported in areas with high incidence of gallbladder cancer, including South America and North India. In developed countries, including the United States, most cases of gallbladder cancer are found incidentally after cholecystectomy. While incidental gallbladder cancer is seen in less than 2% of the routine cholecystectomies done for benign disease, it accounts for more than 50% of all gallbladder cancer diagnosis [7, 8]. The current indications for cholecystectomy in asymptomatic patients have partly been dictated by the presence of risk factors predictive of malignancy. These include patient age more than 60 years with GB polyp less than 10 mm, history of primary sclerosing cholangitis and presence of GB polyp, Asian race, GB wall thickening more than 4 mm, and polyp more than 10 mm [9, 10].

2.2 Imaging

Imaging plays an important role in diagnosing a gallbladder cancer. Ultrasound is the first imaging modality used for gallbladder pathologies. It comes with the advantage of lack of ionizing-radiation exposure, cost-effectiveness, and real-time imaging of the gallbladder (e.g., assessment of intraluminal mass mobility). Ultrasound findings of gallbladder wall thickening, mass, or polyp (measuring more than 10 mm in size) are most suggestive of malignancy [11, 12]. The presence of gallstones and the absence of pericholecystic fluid as seen with acute cholecystitis—in the presence of asymmetric gallbladder thickening—is associated with an increased risk of GBCa [11]. However, routine transabdominal ultrasound is hindered by the observer bias as well as by the negative impact of body habitus and bowel interposition. In recent years, advancement in ultrasound using contrast-enhanced ultrasound imaging (CEUS) and high-resolution ultrasound (HRUS), have greatly enhanced the ability of ultrasound to differentiate between benign and malignant diseases [13, 14]. Endoscopic ultrasound (EUS) is increasingly utilized to improve diagnosis of gallbladder neoplasms. EUS may have a theoretical advantage over traditional transabdominal ultrasound, as it utilizes higher frequency waves and benefits from reduced intervening tissue between the probe and the target of interest [14, 15]. However, direct comparison of endoscopic ultrasound (EUS) and high-resolution transabdominal ultrasound has shown similar rates of diagnosis of gallbladder cancer and neoplastic polyps, with no added benefits obtained by EUS [16, 17]. With these findings, the non-invasive aspect of HRUS makes it preferable over an EUS.

Cross sectional gallbladder imaging may be performed with computed tomography (CT) or magnetic resonance imaging (MRI). Common CT imaging findings for GBCa include GB wall thickening, evidence of an isolated hypodense intraluminal mass, GB wall calcification, and porcelain GB. CT imaging is also especially helpful in identifying infiltration of surrounding organs, LN involvement, peritoneal nodules, and distant metastasis [18, 19]. MRI of the abdomen can also be used to diagnose GBCa, which is seen as an irregular, hypointense lesion on T1-weighted images and hyperintense lesion on T2-weighted images. GBCa often demonstrates early enhancement during MRI performed with gadolinium contrast [20, 21].

GBCa is an FDG-avid malignancy, and thus can be diagnosed with a PET (positron emission tomography) scan [22]. Nonetheless, the low negative predictive value of this test limits its utility [23]. However, the application of FDG PET in the evaluation of residual disease after diagnosis of incidental gallbladder cancer is increasing. While CT scan is the primary imaging to evaluate residual disease, PET has been shown to detect residual disease and LN metastasis in patients with otherwise normal CT scans, in about 25% of the patients [24, 25].

Diagnostic laparoscopy plays a paramount role in confirming pre-operative imaging findings with high applicability in identifying peritoneal disease and/or disseminated solid organ disease. Diagnostic laparoscopy has been shown to identify occult disseminated disease in more than 25% patients of GBCa, who are otherwise found to have localized disease on imaging studies [26]. However, this rate is much lower in patients with incidental GBCa, with benefits noted only in patients with T3/T4 tumors, positive resection margin and poor differentiation on final histopathology evaluation [27].

2.3 Biopsy

Biopsy of suspicious gallbladder masses is not recommended, due to fear of tumor dissemination and bile peritonitis. While previous studies have noted transhepatic route to be safer in terms of GB perforation and peritonitis, the concern for tumor seeding remains. Current NCCN guidelines recommend against biopsy and recommend resection of suspicious masses [28]. Biopsy is however required for patients with unresectable disease to establish diagnosis prior to starting treatment. This has been done percutaneously, laparoscopically or via EUS, however, a core biopsy is preferred for diagnosis [28–30]. Bile cytology obtained through ERCP has also been used to identify GBCa in patients with suspicious lesions. However, recent studies investigating the potential role of liquid biopsy of the bile to identify tumor DNA reported higher predictive value than bile cytology in identifying GBCa [31]. None of these methods are currently indicated in patients who have a potentially resectable tumor and are good surgical candidates.

2.4 Tumor markers

Various tumor markers have been evaluated for gallbladder cancer, and currently, the most used tumor marker in clinical practice is CA19-9. The other tumor markers include CA242, CEA and CA125 [32]. While none of these markers are diagnostic, or specific to GBCa, their levels alone or in combination have been shown to have prognostic implications and may be used to monitor response to therapy [32, 33].

In addition to the tumor markers, various other hematological markers have been shown to have diagnostic and prognostic importance in GBCa. Inflammatory markers have been shown to have prognostic significance with neutrophil-lymphocyte ratio, and platelet-lymphocyte ratio negatively impacting survival and monocyte-lymphocyte ratio predicting response to chemotherapy [34–36]. Recent studies also note the prognostic potential of red cell distribution width and calreticulin in predicting tumor burden [37, 38].

Additionally liquid biopsies identifying circulating free DNA (cf-DNA) and micro-RNA (miRNA) have been shown to have both diagnostic as well as prognostic potential [39, 40]. Identification of certain miRNA mutations may also guide therapeutic interventions [41].

3. Incidental gallbladder cancer and determinants of surgical resection

Incidental GB cancer identified on pathology after routine cholecystectomy, accounts for more than half of the cases of GBCa [7, 8]. Evaluation and management of patients with incidental GBCa is vastly different from patients diagnosed pre-operatively. Since incidental GBCa are identified on pathological evaluation of grossly benign gallbladders, they are identified at an earlier stage and often with no surrounding invasion. As such, patients with incidental GBCa have increased rates of complete resection and better survival than patients who are diagnosed with GBCa pre-operatively [42]. **Table 1** depicts the most recent tumor staging by the AJCC 8th edition classification.

Pathological evaluation of the operative specimen, importantly the depth of invasion (T-stage), involvement of cystic duct margin and in some cases involvement of hepatic or peritoneal surface of the gallbladder, ultimately dictates further management. Re-resection is warranted in most patients to excise residual disease or to obtain adequate margins [8]. Approximately 75% of patients with incidental GBCa—for whom re-resection is performed—demonstrate residual disease which is an independent predictor of poor prognosis. A noteworthy exception—where re-resection is not recommended- is represented by patients with T1a tumors confined to the mucosa—where a simple cholecystectomy is considered an oncologically adequate resection. In addition, resection is not recommended for T4 tumors which are unresectable due to loco-regional invasion and for patients with distant metastatic disease [44, 45]. Re-resection is warranted once the cancer invades through the muscular layer. It is typically described as hepatectomy of segment 4b and 5 with lymphadenectomy of at least six lymph nodes and is associated with improved disease-free survival and overall survival in patients with T1b, T2 and T3 tumors [46, 47]. T2 tumors, where cancer invades the peri-muscular connective tissue without invading the serosa, have been a great area of interest. In this group of patients, the location of the tumor, specifically hepatic surface versus peritoneal surface, has been shown to significantly impact recurrence rates and overall survival [48]. This led to the modification of the

	Stage	Description
T-stage	Tx	Primary tumor cannot be assessed
	T0	No evidence of primary tumor
	T1a	Tumor invades the lamina propria
	T1b	Tumor invades the muscular layer
	T2a	Tumor involves perimuscular connective tissue on the peritoneal side without involving the serosa
	T2b	Tumor involves perimuscular connective tissue on the hepatic side without extension into the liver
	T3	Tumor perforates the serosa (visceral peritoneum) or invades the liver and/or invades one of the adjacent structures or organs (stomach, duodenum, colon, pancreas, omentum, extrahepatic bile duct)
	T4	Tumor invades the main portal vein or hepatic artery or invades two or more extrahepatic structures
N-stage	Nx	Regional lymph nodes cannot be assessed
	N0	No regional lymph nodes
	N1	Metastasis to 1-3 regional lymph nodes
	N2	Metastasis to 4 or more regional lymph nodes
M-stage	M0	No distant metastasis
	M1	Distant metastasis present

T: Tumor; N: Nodal; and M: Metastasis.

Table 1.
TNM staging of gallbladder cancer (AJCC 8th edition) [43].

AJCC staging in the 8th edition to subclassify T2 tumors into T2a where the tumor is located on the peritoneal side and T2b where the tumor is located on the hepatic side [43]. Data suggest that T2b tumors have worse prognosis compared to T2a tumors; in addition, some authors reported improved outcomes when T2b tumors are diagnosed pre-operatively (prior to formal oncological resection) compared to patients who undergo re-resection [48, 49]. Recent studies suggest that hepatic resection only impacts survival in patients with T2b tumors but not T2a [50]. However, the later findings need to be further validated, and the current practice continues to include hepatic resection in all T2 tumors.

Lymph node positivity is an important negative prognostic factor in GBCa. While lymph node (LN) involvement is an important prognostic factor of gallbladder cancer, routine cholecystectomy specimens do not include formal lymphadenectomy [51]. Routine cholecystectomy occasionally includes excision of the cystic node. The positivity of the cystic node has not been shown to be predictive of loco-regional disease, nor is predictive of survival in patients with GBCa [52]. Lymphadenectomy of the pericholedochal, the peri-portal lymph nodes up to the superior-posterior pancreatoduodenal lymph nodes is recommended for complete oncological resection [29]. The presence of positive lymph nodes around the aorta, celiac axis or the SMA constitutes a very poor prognostic factor, with 0% survival noted at 5 years [53]. CBD resection does not improve the quality of the lymph node dissection nor the lymph node yield [54]. In addition, various studies have led to the determination of what constitutes an adequate lymphadenectomy for staging purpose and the current recommendation is for a minimum harvest of six lymph nodes [43]. Bile duct resection is not routinely recommended for gallbladder cancer unless a positive cystic duct margin is noted on final pathology [45].

Residual disease is another important predictor of prognosis in patients with GBCa. Found in more than half of the patients with incidental GBCa, it represents an independent poor prognostic factor, with survival rates similar to patients with metastatic disease [55]. However, recent studies from Japan suggest that the location of residual disease may impact prognosis, with disease in the extrahepatic bile duct or distant sites having worse prognosis compared to disease in the gallbladder bed [56]. While some residual disease may be identified on imaging, specifically PET CT, there are now attempts to develop scoring systems that utilize tumor stage and grade to predict residual disease in patients with GBCa [57].

Lymphovascular invasion and perineural invasion noted in the pathological specimen are also poor prognostic factors [58, 59]. Despite their impact on survival the presence of residual disease, lymphovascular invasion and perineural invasion have no impact on the decision-making for re-resection versus systemic therapy in patients with GBCa. Current attempts on developing additional scoring systems inclusive of these factors remain modest at best [60].

Timing to definitive surgery is a very important determinant of prognosis. Most studies suggest the best outcomes are noted in patients who undergo re-resection between 4 and 8 weeks after the initial cholecystectomy [61].

Intra-operative diagnosis of gallbladder cancer—when resectable—may be ideal, as it would allow the surgeon to perform radical resection during the primary surgery. However multiple concerns remain regarding this approach. Frozen section analysis of suspicious gallbladder lesions remains inconsistent with false positive and false negative results seen in up to 25% of the patients [62]. Additionally, the identification of tumor at the cystic duct margin, which would mandate the need for further biliary duct resection, may be inaccurate in many cases [63]. Thus, current practice for patients undergoing routine cholecystectomy with concerning intra-operative findings remains final histopathology based treatment planning.

4. Systemic therapy in gallbladder cancer

Gallbladder cancer is an aggressive malignancy with early recurrence and metastasis even after complete surgical resection. There is an unmet need for effective systemic therapy and reliable biomarkers specifically for GBCa. Due to the rarity of this disease, most studies investigating systemic therapeutic options often encompass all biliary tract malignancies—including intra and extrahepatic cholangiocarcinoma—which have distinct genetic features and clinical behaviors thus confounding data interpretation and applicability.

4.1 Neoadjuvant therapy

While surgical resection is the mainstay of treatment of GBCa, the high rate of early recurrence after complete resection supports the undeniable need for more effective patient selection strategies for surgical resection and systemic perioperative therapy. Peri-operative therapy and multimodality treatments have been shown to improve outcomes in patients with extrahepatic biliary tract cancers including GBCa [64]. While neoadjuvant therapy has been advantageous in patients with locally advanced disease, there is mounting interest in the use of chemotherapy even in patients with resectable disease [65, 66]. However, data to support this approach are limited, and mostly obtained from studies encompassing all biliary tract cancers, with limited dedicated studies focusing solely on GBCa.

Neoadjuvant chemotherapy for GBCa has evolved significantly over the last two decades. Currently the first line neoadjuvant therapy consists of Gemcitabine-Cisplatin (Gem-Cis) based chemotherapy, which has been shown to improve overall survival and progression free survival compared to both gemcitabine and 5-Flurouracil (5-FU) based chemotherapy [67, 68]. Recently, higher response rates—up to 40–50%—were reported with the use of combination chemotherapy by combining "gemcitabine- nab-paclitaxel- cisplatin" [69]. Additional studies conducted on patients who have disease refractory to Gem-Cis have shown improved progression free survival with the administration of FOLFOX or FOLFIRI, justifying the use of these regimens as second line therapy in GBCa [70, 71] (**Table 2**).

There is currently no clear evidence supporting the use of neoadjuvant chemoradiation in patients with GBCa [72]. However, a phase III randomized trial—POLCAGB—is currently underway comparing the survival outcomes of neoadjuvant chemotherapy versus chemoradiotherapy in patients with GBCa [73].

Immunotherapy has been shown to improve response to chemotherapy and impact survival in patients with GBCa in patients with locally advanced—unresectable or metastatic disease. PD-L1 is a known target for immunotherapy that is present in about a quarter of pathological specimens of biliary tract cancer [74, 75]. Studies have shown improved response rates to neoadjuvant therapy when PD-L1 inhibitor, Durvalumab is combined with Gem-Cis [76]. The TOPAZ-1 trial confirmed the safety and efficacy of Durvalumab plus Gem-Cis, demonstrating improved overall survival versus placebo plus chemotherapy (estimated 24-month was 24.9% vs. 10.4%). Moreover, it showed improvements in prespecified secondary end points including objective response rate up to 26.7% vs. 18.7% (OR 1.6; 95% CI, 1.11–2.31). It is important to note that the

Publication	Study	Patients	Comparison	Result
Valle et al., 2010 (ABC-02) [68]	RCT	410 (LA, metastatic)	Gemcitabine vs. Gem-Cis	Gem-Cis: Improved OS & PFS
Phelip et al., 2022 (PRODIGE 38 AMEBICA) [67]	RCT	191 (LA, metastatic)	Gem-Cis vs. FOLFIRINOX	No advantage
Shroff et al., 2019 [69]	RCT	62 (LA, metastatic)	Gem-Cis- nab-Paclitaxel vs. Gem-cis	Gem-Cis- nab-Paclitaxel: Improved OS & PFS
Lamarca et al., 2021 (ABC 06) [70]	RCT	162 (LA, metastatic, progression with Gem-Cis)	FOLFOX vs. ASC	FOLFOX: Improved PFS
Yoo et al., 2021 (NIFTY) [71]	RCT	174 (metastatic progression with Gem-Cis)	FOLFIRI vs. 5FU and leucovorin	FOLFIRI: Improved PFS

ABC: advanced biliary cancer; RCT: randomized control trial; Gem-Cis: gemcitabine- cisplatin; LA: locally advanced; FOLFIRINOX: 5-flurouracil- irinotecan-oxaliplatin; FOLFOX: 5-flurouracil-oxaliplatin; FOLFIRI: 5-flurouracil-irinotecan; 5FU: 5-flurouracil; OS: overall survival; and PFS: progression free survival.

Table 2.
Trials evaluating chemotherapy use in gallbladder cancer.

TOPAZ-1 trial was designed to address a locally advanced-unresectable or metastatic population of biliary tract cancer—among which approximately 25% represented GBca—with previously untreated disease but included patients who developed recurrent disease more than 6 months after surgery with curative intent and more than 6 months after the completion of adjuvant therapy [77].

4.2 Adjuvant therapy

Due to the low incidence of GBCa, most of the data on the impact of adjuvant therapy on survival of patients with GBCa are derived from studies done on patients with any biliary tract cancer. While initial randomized control trials with gemcitabine-based adjuvant therapy failed to show a survival benefit in biliary tract cancers, examination of adjuvant capecitabine (BILCAP trial), suggested positive trends towards survival when adjusted for nodal positivity and tumor grade [78–80]. These studies also prompted dedicated examination of patients with GBCa. Retrospective analysis of large cohorts, including two studies that utilized National Cancer Database and a subsequent meta-analysis of more than 20,000 patients have shown an association between adjuvant chemotherapy and prolonged survival in patients with GBCa, especially in the presence of node positive disease [81–84].

There is also an increased interest in the use of adjuvant chemoradiotherapy in gallbladder cancer. Recent studies including propensity matched analysis of patients receiving adjuvant chemoradiotherapy versus chemotherapy have noted improved survival and reduced local recurrence associated with the use of adjuvant chemoradiation. These findings are especially noted in patients with tumor stage T2 or lymph node positive disease [85, 86]. In addition, a secondary analysis of the phase II intergroup trial, SWOG S0809—that evaluated adjuvant capecitabine and gemcitabine followed by radiotherapy and concurrent capecitabine—demonstrated improved OS in patients with extrahepatic cholangiocarcinoma and GBCa compared to historical controls. Furthermore, the data suggested that adjuvant chemoradiation positively impacted local control in patients with node positive disease [87].

4.3 Peri-operative chemotherapy

There is now a great interest in the use of peri-operative therapy in patients with incidental GBCa (i.e., prior to formal oncological resection in patients who are diagnosed with incidental GBCa after a cholecystectomy). It may be hypothesized that timing of systemic therapy prior to formal resection would allow downstaging of the residual disease, allowing complete resection of the tumor. While no definitive data exist to suggest the superiority of either regimen (i.e., peri-operative versus adjuvant) there are currently two randomized control trials underway to ascertain the merits of the two approaches. Both the OPT-IN trial and the ACO-GAIN trial are examining the difference in oncological outcomes of patients treated with peri-operative gemcitabine- cisplatin therapy compared to those who undergo radical resection without any intervening systemic therapy [88, 89].

5. Surgical resection of GBCa

All GBCa with T-stage including T1b to T3 warrant a radical cholecystectomy after having ascertained the absence of distal lymphadenopathy (i.e., periaortic, celiac, and retropancreatic) and metastatic disease. Similar to the operative principles used in patients undergoing re-resection, patients diagnosed pre-operatively and those found to have GBCa on intra-operative frozen section should undergo cholecystectomy with hepatic resection of segment 4b and 5, along with lymphadenectomy with bile duct resection reserved only for obtaining negative margins [45]. Additional aspects of the surgery may include bile duct resection, vascular resection and extended hepatectomy, all of which are performed with the single goal of obtaining negative resection margins. There is currently no role of port site resection in patients who were diagnosed following a previous laparoscopic cholecystectomy, as this practice does not impact disease-free or overall survival [90].

Traditionally, the concern for port site seeding, chimney effect and concern for peritoneal dissemination, led to radical cholecystectomy being done as an exclusively open procedure [91–93]. However, studies comparing minimally invasive and open radical cholecystectomies have noted no oncological differences between laparoscopic and open surgery, with improved intra-operative and peri-operative outcomes in patients undergoing laparoscopic resection [94, 95]. Thus this procedure is now performed both laparoscopically and robotically. While most of the data on robotic oncological safety is derived from studies on laparoscopic radical cholecystectomy, there is an increasing trend of utilization of the robotic platform for this surgical procedure [96, 97].

6. Conclusion

Gallbladder cancer, although rare, is an aggressive malignancy and the most common biliary tract cancer. With the increased cholecystectomy rate, most patients in the western world are diagnosed incidentally. Pathological evaluation of the gallbladder not only establishes diagnosis, but also guides further treatment planning, based on the accurate knowledge of the T-stage and of the cystic duct margin. The early systemic recurrence and poor overall survival—even after complete resection—warrant the use of multimodality treatment with chemotherapy and immunotherapy. Systemic therapy is currently the first line treatment in patients unable to undergo surgical resection, moreover, it is increasingly being advocated in the neoadjuvant and perioperative period to improve resection rates and possibly disease-free survival.

Conflict of interest

The authors declare no conflict of interest.

Author details

Asmita Chopra[1] and Alessandro Paniccia[2*]

1 Department of Surgery, University of Toledo, Toledo, OH, USA

2 Department of Surgery, University of Pittsburgh, Pittsburgh, PA, USA

*Address all correspondence to: panicciaa2@upmc.edu

References

[1] Survival rates in Gallbladder cancer. American Cancer Society. Available from: https://www.cancer.org/cancer/gallbladder-cancer/detection-diagnosis-staging/survival-rates.html#references [Accessed: August 7, 2022]

[2] Lazcano-Ponce EC, Miquel JF, Muñoz N, et al. Epidemiology and molecular pathology of gallbladder cancer. CA: A Cancer Journal for Clinicians. 2001;**51**(6):349-364. DOI: 10.3322/canjclin.51.6.349

[3] Randi G, Franceschi S, La Vecchia C. Gallbladder cancer worldwide: Geographical distribution and risk factors. International Journal of Cancer. 2006;**118**(7):1591-1602. DOI: 10.1002/ijc.21683

[4] Hundal R, Shaffer EA. Gallbladder cancer: Epidemiology and outcome. Clinical Epidemiology. 2014;**6**:99-109. DOI: 10.2147/CLEP.S37357

[5] Henley SJ, Weir HK, Jim MA, Watson M, Richardson LC. Gallbladder cancer incidence and mortality, United States 1999-2011. Cancer Epidemiology, Biomarkers & Prevention. 2015;**24**(9):1319-1326. DOI: 10.1158/1055-9965.EPI-15-0199

[6] Kuipers H, de Bitter TJJ, de Boer MT, van der Post RS, Nijkamp MW, de Reuver PR, et al. Gallbladder cancer: Current insights in genetic alterations and their possible therapeutic implications. Cancers (Basel). 2021;**13**(21):5257. DOI: 10.3390/cancers13215257

[7] Kellil T, Chaouch MA, Aloui E, Tormane MA, Taieb SK, Noomen F, et al. Incidence and preoperative predictor factors of gallbladder cancer before laparoscopic cholecystectomy: A systematic review. Journal of Gastrointestinal Cancer. 2021;**52**(1): 68-72. DOI: 10.1007/s12029-020-00524-7

[8] Cavallaro A, Piccolo G, Di Vita M, Zanghì A, Cardì F, Di Mattia P, et al. Managing the incidentally detected gallbladder cancer: Algorithms and controversies. International Journal of Surgery. 2014;**12**(Suppl 2):S108-S119. DOI: 10.1016/j.ijsu.2014.08.367

[9] Muszynska C, Nilsson J, Lundgren L, Lindell G, Andersson R, Sandström P, et al. A risk score model to predict incidental gallbladder cancer in patients scheduled for cholecystectomy. American Journal of Surgery. 2020;**220**(3):741-744. DOI: 10.1016/j.amjsurg.2020.01.039

[10] Aziz H, Hewitt DB, Pawlik TM. Critical analysis of the updated guidelines for management of gallbladder polyps. Annals of Surgical Oncology. 2022;**29**(6):3363-3365. DOI: 10.1245/s10434-022-11701-2

[11] Goussous N, Maqsood H, Patel K, Ferdosi H, Muhammad N, Sill AM, et al. Clues to predict incidental gallbladder cancer. Hepatobiliary & Pancreatic Diseases International. 2018;**17**(2):149-154. DOI: 10.1016/j.hbpd.2018.02.001

[12] Zevallos Maldonado C, Ruiz Lopez MJ, Gonzalez Valverde FM, Alarcon Soldevilla F, Pastor Quirante F, Garcia MV. Ultrasound findings associated to gallbladder carcinoma. Cirugía Española. 2014;**92**(5):348-355. DOI: 10.1016/j.ciresp.2012.10.007

[13] Serra C, Felicani C, Mazzotta E, Gabusi V, Grasso V, De Cinque A, et al. CEUS in the differential diagnosis between biliary sludge, benign lesions and malignant lesions. Journal of

Ultrasound. 2018;**21**(2):119-126. DOI: 10.1007/s40477-018-0286-5

[14] Yu MH, Kim YJ, Park HS, Jung SI. Benign gallbladder diseases: Imaging techniques and tips for differentiating with malignant gallbladder diseases. World Journal of Gastroenterology. 2020;**26**(22):2967-2986. DOI: 10.3748/wjg.v26.i22.2967

[15] Kim HJ, Park JH, Park DI, Cho YK, Sohn CI, Jeon WK, et al. Clinical usefulness of endoscopic ultrasonography in the differential diagnosis of gallbladder wall thickening. Digestive Diseases and Sciences. 2012;**57**(2):508-515. DOI: 10.1007/s10620-011-1870-0

[16] Wennmacker SZ, Lamberts MP, Di Martino M, Drenth JP, Gurusamy KS, van Laarhoven CJ. Transabdominal ultrasound and endoscopic ultrasound for diagnosis of gallbladder polyps. Cochrane Database of Systematic Reviews. 2018;**8**(8):CD012233. DOI: 10.1002/14651858.CD012233.pub2

[17] Lee JS, Kim JH, Kim YJ, Ryu JK, Kim YT, Lee JY, et al. Diagnostic accuracy of transabdominal high-resolution US for staging gallbladder cancer and differential diagnosis of neoplastic polyps compared with EUS. European Radiology. 2017;**27**(7):3097-3103. DOI: 10.1007/s00330-016-4646-2

[18] Han H, Han J. Value of multislice spiral CT in differential diagnosis of thick-wall gallbladder carcinoma and chronic cholecystitis. Contrast Media & Molecular Imaging. 2022;**2022**:5459779. DOI: 10.1155/2022/5459779

[19] Zhang L, Hou C, Chen M, Guo L, Xu Z, Wang L, et al. Tumour radiological appearance evaluated by enhanced CT correlates with tumour progression and survival in curable gallbladder cancer. European Journal of Surgical Oncology. 2020;**46**(11):2099-2105. DOI: 10.1016/j.ejso.2020.07.006

[20] Tan CH, Lim KS. MRI of gallbladder cancer. Diagnostic and Interventional Radiology. 2013;**19**(4):312-319. DOI: 10.5152/dir.2013.044

[21] Gore RM, Thakrar KH, Newmark GM, Mehta UK, Berlin JW. Gallbladder imaging. Gastroenterology Clinics of North America. 2010;**39**(2):265-287. DOI: 10.1016/j.gtc.2010.02.009

[22] Ramos-Font C, Gómez-Rio M, Rodríguez-Fernández A, Jiménez-Heffernan A, Sánchez Sánchez R, Llamas-Elvira JM. Ability of FDG-PET/CT in the detection of gallbladder cancer. Journal of Surgical Oncology. 2014;**109**(3):218-224. DOI: 10.1002/jso.23476

[23] Lee SW, Kim HJ, Park JH, Park DI, Cho YK, Sohn CI, et al. Clinical usefulness of 18F-FDG PET-CT for patients with gallbladder cancer and cholangiocarcinoma. Journal of Gastroenterology. 2010;**45**(5):560-566. DOI: 10.1007/s00535-009-0188-6

[24] Shukla PJ, Barreto SG, Arya S, Shrikhande SV, Hawaldar R, Purandare N, et al. Does PET-CT scan have a role prior to radical re-resection for incidental gallbladder cancer? HPB: The Official Journal of the International Hepato Pancreato Biliary Association. 2008;**10**(6):439-445. DOI: 10.1080/13651820802286910

[25] Albazaz R, Patel CN, Chowdhury FU, Scarsbrook AF. Clinical impact of FDG PET-CT on management decisions for patients with primary biliary tumors. Insights Into Imaging. 2013;**4**(5):691-700. DOI: 10.1007/s13244-013-0268-2

[26] Tian Y, Liu L, Yeolkar NV, Shen F, Li J, He Z. Diagnostic role of staging laparoscopy in a subset of biliary cancers: A meta-analysis. ANZ Journal of Surgery. 2017;**87**(1-2):22-27. DOI: 10.1111/ans.13762

[27] Butte JM, Gönen M, Allen PJ, D'Angelica MI, Kingham TP, Fong Y, et al. The role of laparoscopic staging in patients with incidental gallbladder cancer. HPB: The Official Journal of the International Hepato Pancreato Biliary Association. 2011;**13**(7):463-472. DOI: 10.1111/j.1477-2574.2011.00325.x

[28] National Comprehensive Cancer Network. Hepatobiliary Cancer (Version 2.2022). Available from: https://www.nccn.org/professionals/physician_gls/pdf/hepatobiliary.pdf

[29] Zargar SA, Khuroo MS, Mahajan R, Jan GM, Shah P. US-guided fine-needle aspiration biopsy of gallbladder masses. Radiology. 1991;**179**(1):275-278. DOI: 10.1148/radiology.179.1.2006291

[30] Kang SH, Joo JS, Kim SH, Kim KH, Lee ES. EUS-guided fine-needle biopsy of gallbladder polypoid lesions. VideoGIE. 2020;**5**(4):151-153. DOI: 10.1016/j.vgie.2019.12.004

[31] Kinugasa H, Nouso K, Ako S, Dohi C, Matsushita H, Matsumoto K, et al. Liquid biopsy of bile for the molecular diagnosis of gallbladder cancer. Cancer Biology & Therapy. 2018;**19**(10):934-938. DOI: 10.1080/15384047.2018.1456604

[32] Rana S, Dutta U, Kochhar R, Rana SV, Gupta R, Pal R, et al. Evaluation of CA 242 as a tumor marker in gallbladder cancer. Journal of Gastrointestinal Cancer. 2012;**43**(2):267-271. DOI: 10.1007/s12029-011-9288-7

[33] Wang YF, Feng FL, Zhao XH, Ye ZX, Zeng HP, Li Z, et al. Combined detection tumor markers for diagnosis and prognosis of gallbladder cancer. World Journal of Gastroenterology. 2014;**20**(14):4085-4092. DOI: 10.3748/wjg.v20.i14.4085

[34] Tao Z, Li SX, Cui X, et al. The prognostic value of preoperative inflammatory indexes in gallbladder carcinoma with hepatic involvement. Cancer Biomarkers. 2018;**22**(3):551-557. DOI: 10.3233/CBM-181230

[35] Zhang Y, Jiang C, Li J, Sun J, Qu X. Prognostic significance of preoperative neutrophil/lymphocyte ratio and platelet/lymphocyte ratio in patients with gallbladder carcinoma. Clinical & Translational Oncology. 2015;**17**(10):810-818. DOI: 10.1007/s12094-015-1310-2

[36] Choi YH, Lee JW, Lee SH, et al. A high monocyte-to-lymphocyte ratio predicts poor prognosis in patients with advanced gallbladder cancer receiving chemotherapy. Cancer Epidemiology, Biomarkers & Prevention. 2019;**28**(6):1045-1051. DOI: 10.1158/1055-9965.EPI-18-1066

[37] Xie Y, Zhang L, Zhan L. Can we assess the advancements of gallbladder cancer using red blood cell distribution width? Medicine (Baltimore). 2019;**98**(51):e18364. DOI: 10.1097/MD.0000000000018364

[38] Ye J, Qi L, Du Z, et al. Calreticulin: A potential diagnostic and therapeutic biomarker in gallbladder cancer. Aging (Albany NY). 2021;**13**(4):5607-5620. DOI: 10.18632/aging.202488

[39] Kumari S, Tewari S, Husain N, et al. Quantification of circulating free DNA as a diagnostic marker in gall bladder cancer. Pathology Oncology Research. 2017;**23**(1):91-97. DOI: 10.1007/s12253-016-0087-0

[40] Tekcham DS, Tiwari PK. Non-coding RNAs as emerging molecular targets of gallbladder cancer. Gene. 2016;**588**(1):79-85. DOI: 10.1016/j.gene.2016.04.047

[41] Yang G, Lu Z, Meng F, et al. Circulating miR-141 as a potential biomarker for diagnosis, prognosis and therapeutic targets in gallbladder cancer. Scientific Reports. 2022;**12**(1):10072. DOI: 10.1038/s41598-022-13430-8

[42] Fong Y, Jarnagin W, Blumgart LH. Gallbladder cancer: Comparison of patients presenting initially for definitive operation with those presenting after prior noncurative intervention. Annals of Surgery. 2000;**232**(4):557-569. DOI: 10.1097/00000658-200010000-00011

[43] Amin MB, Greene FL, Edge SB, et al. The eighth edition AJCC cancer staging manual. CA: A Cancer Journal for Clinicians. 2017;**67**(2):93-99. DOI: 10.3322/caac.21388

[44] Cherkassky L, D'Angelica M. Gallbladder cancer: Managing the incidental diagnosis. Surgical Oncology Clinics of North America. 2019;**28**(4):619-630. DOI: 10.1016/j.soc.2019.06.005

[45] Aloia TA, Járufe N, Javle M, Maithel SK, Roa JC, Adsay V, et al. Gallbladder cancer: Expert consensus statement. HPB: The Official Journal of the International Hepato Pancreato Biliary Association. 2015;**17**(8):681-690. DOI: 10.1111/hpb.12444

[46] Fuks D, Regimbeau JM, Le Treut YP, Bachellier P, Raventos A, Pruvot FR, et al. Incidental gallbladder cancer by the AFC-GBC-2009 study group. World Journal of Surgery. 2011;**35**(8):1887-1897. DOI: 10.1007/s00268-011-1134-3

[47] Hari DM, Howard JH, Leung AM, Chui CG, Sim MS, Bilchik AJ. A 21-year analysis of stage I gallbladder carcinoma: Is cholecystectomy alone adequate? HPB: The Official Journal of the International Hepato Pancreato Biliary Association. 2013;**15**(1):40-48. DOI: 10.1111/j.1477-2574.2012.00559.x

[48] Kim WJ, Lim TW, Park PJ, Choi SB, Kim WB. Clinicopathological differences in T2 gallbladder cancer according to tumor location. Cancer Control. 2020;**27**(1):1073274820915514. DOI: 10.1177/1073274820915514

[49] Vega EA, Vinuela E, Okuno M, Joechle K, Sanhueza M, Diaz C, et al. Incidental versus non-incidental gallbladder cancer: Index cholecystectomy before oncologic re-resection negatively impacts survival in T2b tumors. HPB: The Official Journal of the International Hepato Pancreato Biliary Association. 2019;**21**(8):1046-1056. DOI: 10.1016/j.hpb.2018.12.006

[50] Alrawashdeh W, Kamarajah SK, Gujjuri RR, Cambridge WA, Shrikhande SV, Wei AC, et al. Systematic review and meta-analysis of survival outcomes in T2a and T2b gallbladder cancers. HPB: The Official Journal of the International Hepato Pancreato Biliary Association. 2022;**24**(6):789-796. DOI: 10.1016/j.hpb.2021.12.019

[51] Bartlett DL, Fong Y, Fortner JG, Brennan MF, Blumgart LH. Long-term results after resection for gallbladder cancer. Implications for staging and management. Annals of Surgery. 1996;**224**(5):639-646. DOI: 10.1097/00000658-199611000-00008

[52] Vega EA, Vinuela E, Yamashita S, Sanhueza M, Cavada G, Diaz C, et al. Extended lymphadenectomy is required for incidental gallbladder cancer independent of cystic duct lymph node status. Journal of Gastrointestinal

Surgery. 2018;**22**(1):43-51. DOI: 10.1007/s11605-017-3507-x

[53] Shimada H, Endo I, Togo S, Nakano A, Izumi T, Nakagawara G. The role of lymph node dissection in the treatment of gallbladder carcinoma. Cancer. 1997;**79**(5):892-899. DOI: 10.1002/(sici)1097-0142(19970301)79:5<892::aid-cncr4>3.0.co;2-e

[54] Gani F, Buettner S, Margonis GA, Ethun CG, Poultsides G, Tran T, et al. Assessing the impact of common bile duct resection in the surgical management of gallbladder cancer. Journal of Surgical Oncology. 2016;**114**(2):176-180. DOI: 10.1002/jso.24283

[55] Butte JM, Kingham TP, Gönen M, D'Angelica MI, Allen PJ, Fong Y, et al. Residual disease predicts outcomes after definitive resection for incidental gallbladder cancer. Journal of the American College of Surgeons. 2014;**219**(3):416-429. DOI: 10.1016/j.jamcollsurg.2014.01.069

[56] Ando T, Sakata J, Nomura T, Takano K, Takizawa K, Miura K, et al. Anatomic location of residual disease after initial cholecystectomy independently determines outcomes after re-resection for incidental gallbladder cancer. Langenbeck's Archives of Surgery. 2021;**406**(5):1521-1532. DOI: 10.1007/s00423-021-02165-1

[57] Ethun CG, Postlewait LM, Le N, Pawlik TM, Buettner S, Poultsides G, et al. A novel pathology-based preoperative risk score to predict locoregional residual and distant disease and survival for incidental gallbladder cancer: A 10-institution study from the U.S. extrahepatic biliary malignancy consortium. Annals of Surgical Oncology. 2017;**24**(5):1343-1350. DOI: 10.1245/s10434-016-5637-x

[58] Dominguez DA, Aversa JG, Hagerty BL, Diggs LP, Raoof M, Davis JL, et al. Prognostic impact of lymphovascular invasion in pT1-T3 gallbladder adenocarcinoma. Journal of Surgical Oncology. 2020;**122**(7):1401-1408. DOI: 10.1002/jso.26160

[59] Yamaguchi R, Nagino M, Oda K, Kamiya J, Uesaka K, Nimura Y. Perineural invasion has a negative impact on survival of patients with gallbladder carcinoma. The British Journal of Surgery. 2002;**89**(9):1130-1136. DOI: 10.1046/j.1365-2168.2002.02184.x

[60] Creasy JM, Goldman DA, Gonen M, Dudeja V, Askan G, Basturk O, et al. Predicting residual disease in incidental gallbladder cancer: Risk stratification for modified treatment strategies. Journal of Gastrointestinal Surgery. 2017;**21**(8):1254-1261. DOI: 10.1007/s11605-017-3436-8

[61] Ethun CG, Postlewait LM, Le N, Pawlik TM, Buettner S, Poultsides G, et al. Association of optimal time interval to re-resection for incidental gallbladder cancer with overall survival: A multi-institution analysis from the US extrahepatic biliary malignancy consortium. JAMA Surgery. 2017;**152**(2):143-149. DOI: 10.1001/jamasurg.2016.3642

[62] Yamaguchi K, Chijiiwa K, Saiki S, Shimizu S, Tsuneyoshi M, Tanaka M. Reliability of frozen section diagnosis of gallbladder tumor for detecting carcinoma and depth of its invasion. Journal of Surgical Oncology. 1997;**65**(2):132-136. DOI: 10.1002/(sici)1096-9098(199706)65:2<132::aid-jso11>3.0.co;2-7

[63] Yamaguchi K, Shirahane K, Nakamura M, et al. Frozen section and permanent diagnoses of the bile duct margin in gallbladder and bile duct

cancer. HPB: The Official Journal of the International Hepato Pancreato Biliary Association. 2005;**7**(2):135-138. DOI: 10.1080/13651820510028873

[64] Patkar S, Ostwal V, Ramaswamy A, Engineer R, Chopra S, Shetty N, et al. Emerging role of multimodality treatment in gall bladder cancer: Outcomes following 510 consecutive resections in a tertiary referral center. Journal of Surgical Oncology. 2018;**117**(3):372-379. DOI: 10.1002/jso.24837

[65] Chaudhari VA, Ostwal V, Patkar S, Sahu A, Toshniwal A, Ramaswamy A, et al. Outcome of neoadjuvant chemotherapy in "locally advanced/borderline resectable" gallbladder cancer: The need to define indications. HPB: The Official Journal of the International Hepato Pancreato Biliary Association. 2018;**20**(9):841-847. DOI: 10.1016/j.hpb.2018.03.008

[66] Sirohi B, Mitra A, Jagannath P, Singh A, Ramadvar M, Kulkarni S, et al. Neoadjuvant chemotherapy in patients with locally advanced gallbladder cancer. Future Oncology. 2015;**11**(10):1501-1509. DOI: 10.2217/fon.14.308

[67] Phelip JM, Desrame J, Edeline J, et al. Modified FOLFIRINOX versus CISGEM chemotherapy for patients with advanced biliary tract cancer (PRODIGE 38 AMEBICA): A randomized phase II study. Journal of Clinical Oncology. 2022;**40**(3):262-271. DOI: 10.1200/JCO.21.00679

[68] Valle J, Wasan H, Palmer DH, et al. Cisplatin plus gemcitabine versus gemcitabine for biliary tract cancer. The New England Journal of Medicine. 2010;**362**(14):1273-1281. DOI: 10.1056/NEJMoa0908721

[69] Shroff RT, Jayle MM, Xiao L, et al. Gemcitabine, cisplatin, and nab-paclitaxel for the treatment of advanced biliary tract cancers: A phase 2 clinical trial. JAMA Oncology. 2019;**5**(6):824-830. DOI: 10.100/jamaoncol.2019.0270

[70] Lamarca A, Palmer DH, Wasan HS, et al. Second-line FOLFOX chemotherapy versus active symptom control for advanced biliary tract cancer (ABC-06): A phase 3, open-label, randomized, controlled trial. The Lancet Oncology. 2021;**22**(5):690-701. DOI: 10.1016/S1470-2045(21)00027-9

[71] Yoo C, Kim KP, Jeong JH, et al. Liposomal irinotecan plus fluorouracil and leucovorin versus fluorouracil and leucovorin for metastatic biliary tract cancer after progression on gemcitabine plus cisplatin (NIFTY): A multicentre, open-label, randomized, phase 2b study. The Lancet Oncology. 2021;**22**(11):1560-1572. DOI: 10/1016/S1470-2045(21)00486-1. De

[72] Aretxbala X, Losada H, Mora J, et al. Neoadjuvant chemoradiotherapy in gallbladder cancer. Revista Médica de Chile. 2004;**132**:51-57

[73] Engineer R, Patkar S, Lewis SC, et al. A phase III randomized clinical trial of perioperative therapy (neoadjuvant chemotherapy versus chemoradiotherapy) in locally advanced gallbladder cancers (POLCAGB): Study protocol. BMJ Open. 2019;**9**(6):e028147. DOI: 10.1136/bmjopen-2018-028147

[74] Neyaz A, Husain N, Kumari S, Gupta S, Shukla S, Arshad S, et al. Clinical relevance of PD-L1 expression in gallbladder cancer: A potential target for therapy. Histopathology. 2018;**73**(4):622-633. DOI: 10.1111/his.13669

[75] Rizzo A, Ricci AD, Brandi G. Durvalumab: An investigational anti-PD-L1 antibody for the treatment of biliary tract cancer. Expert Opinion on Investigational

Drugs. 2021;**30**(4):343-350. DOI: 10.1080/13543784.2021.1897102

[76] Oh DY, Lee KH, Lee DW, et al. Gemcitabine and cisplatin plus durvalumab with or without tremelimumab in chemotherapy-naïve patients with advanced biliary tract cancer: An open-label, single-Centre, phase 2 study. Lancet Gastroenterología y Hepatología. 2022;7(6):522-532. DOI: 10.1016/S2468-1253(22)000437

[77] Oh DY, He AR, Qin S, et al. Durvalumab plus gemcitabine and cisplatin in advanced biliary tract cancer. NEJM EVID. 2022;**1**(8). DOI: 10.1056/EVIDoa2200015

[78] Primrose JN, Fox RP, Palmer DH, et al. BILCAP study group. Capecitabine compared with observation in resected biliary tract cancer (BILCAP): A randomised, controlled, multicentre, phase 3 study. The Lancet Oncology. 2019;**20**(5):663-673. DOI: 10.1016/S1470-2045(18)30915-X

[79] Edeline J, Benabdelghani M, Bertaut A, et al. Gemcitabine and oxaliplatin chemotherapy or surveillance in resected biliary tract cancer (PRODIGE 12-ACCORD 18-UNICANCER GI): A randomized phase III study. Journal of Clinical Oncology. 2019;**37**(8):658-667. DOI: 10.1200/JCO.18.00050

[80] Ebata T, Hirano S, Konishi M, Uesaka K, Tsuchiya Y, Ohtsuka M, et al. Randomized clinical trial of adjuvant gemcitabine chemotherapy versus observation in resected bile duct cancer. The British Journal of Surgery. 2018;**105**(3):192-202. DOI: 10.1002/bjs.10776

[81] Tran Cao HS, Zhang Q, Sada YH, Chai C, Curley SA, Massarweh NN. The role of surgery and adjuvant therapy in lymph node-positive cancers of the gallbladder and intrahepatic bile ducts. Cancer. 2018;**124**(1):74-83. DOI: 10.1002/cncr.30968

[82] Bergquist JR, Shah HN, Habermann ED, et al. Adjuvant systemic therapy after resection of node positive gallbladder cancer: Time for a well-designed tiral? (results if a US-national retrospective cohort study). International Journal of Surgery. 2018;**52**:171-179. DOI: 10.1016/j.ijsu.2018.02.052

[83] Hoehn RS, Wima K, Ertel AE, et al. Adjuvant therapy for gallbladder cancer: An analysis of the National Cancer Database. Journal of Gastrointestinal Surgery. 2015;**19**(10):1794-1801. DOI: 1007/s11605-015-2922-0

[84] Ghidini M, Tomasello G, Botticelli A, et al. Adjuvant chemotherapy for resected biliary tract cancers: A systemic review and meta-analysis. HPB: The Official Journal of the International Hepato Pancreato Biliary Association. 2017;**19**(9):741-748. DOI: 10.1016/j.hpb.2017.05.010

[85] Gu B, Qian L, Yu H, et al. Concurrent chemoradiotherapy in curatively resected gallbladder carcinoma: A propensity score-matched analysis. International Journal of Radiation Oncology, Biology, Physics. 2018;**100**(1):138-145. DOI: 10.1016/j.ijrobp.2017.09.029

[86] Kim TG. Patterns of intial failure after resection for gallbladder cancer: Implications for adjuvant radiotherapy. Radiation Oncology Journal. 2017;**35**(4):359-367. DOI: 10.3857/roj.2017.00388

[87] Ben-Josef E, Guthrie KA, El-Khoueiry AB, et al. SWOG S0809: A phase II intergroup trial of adjuvant capecitabine and gemcitabine followed by radiotherapy and concurrent capecitabine in extrahepatic

cholangiocarcinoma and gallbladder carcinoma. Journal of Clinical Oncology. 2015;**33**(24):2617-2622. DOI: 10.1200/JCO.2014.60.2219

[88] Khan TM, Verbus EA, Hong H, Ethun CG, Maithel SK, Hernandez JM. Perioperative versus adjuvant chemotherapy in the Management of Incidentally Found Gallbladder Cancer (OPT-IN). Annals of Surgical Oncology. 2022;**29**(1):37-38. DOI: 10.1245/s10434-021-10277-7

[89] Goetze TO, Bechstein WO, Bankstahl US, Keck T, Königsrainer A, Lang SA, et al. Neoadjuvant chemotherapy with gemcitabine plus cisplatin followed by radical liver resection versus immediate radical liver resection alone with or without adjuvant chemotherapy in incidentally detected gallbladder carcinoma after simple cholecystectomy or in front of radical resection of BTC (ICC/ECC)—A phase III study of the German registry of incidental gallbladder carcinoma platform (GR)- the AIO/CALGP/ACO-GAIN-trial. BMC Cancer. 2020;**20**(1):122. DOI: 10.1186/s12885-020-6610-4

[90] Maker AV, Butte JM, Oxenberg J, Kuk D, Gonen M, Fong Y, et al. Is port site resection necessary in the surgical management of gallbladder cancer? Annals of Surgical Oncology. 2012;**19**(2):409-417. DOI: 10.1245/s10434-011-1850-9

[91] Berger-Richardson D, Chesney TR, Englesakis M, Govindarajan A, Cleary SP, Swallow CJ. Trends in port-site metastasis after laparoscopic resection of incidental gallbladder cancer: A systematic review. Surgery. 2017;**161**(3):618-627. DOI: 10.1016/j.surg.2016.08.007

[92] Lundberg O. Port site metastases after laparoscopic cholecystectomy. The European Journal of Surgery. 2000;**585**:27-30. DOI: 10.1080/110241500750056508

[93] Lundberg O, Kristoffersson A. Port site metastases from gallbladder cancer after laparoscopic cholecystectomy. Results of a Swedish survey and review of published reports. The European Journal of Surgery. 1999;**165**(3):215-222. DOI: 10.1080/110241599750007072

[94] Nag HH, Sachan A, Nekarakanti PK. Laparoscopic versus open extended cholecystectomy with bi-segmentectomy (s4b and s5) in patients with gallbladder cancer. Journal of Minimal Access Surgery. 2021;**17**(1):21-27. DOI: 10.4103/jmas.JMAS_98_19

[95] Dou C, Zhang Y, Liu J, Wei F, Chu H, Han J, et al. Laparoscopy versus laparotomy approach of a radical resection for gallbladder cancer: A retrospective comparative study. Surgical Endoscopy. 2020;**34**(7):2926-2938. DOI: 10.1007/s00464-019-07075-4

[96] Muaddi H, Hafid ME, Choi WJ, Lillie E, de Mestral C, Nathens A, et al. Clinical outcomes of robotic surgery compared to conventional surgical approaches (laparoscopic or open): A systematic overview of reviews. Annals of Surgery. 2021;**273**(3):467-473. DOI: 10.1097/SLA.0000000000003915

[97] AlMasri S, Nassour I, Tohme S, et al. Long-term survival following minimally invasive extended cholecystectomy for gallbladder cancer: A 7-year experience from the National Cancer Database. [published online ahead of print, 2020 Jun 12]. Journal of Surgical Oncology. 2020;**10**. DOI: 10.1002/jso.26062

Section 5

Bile Duct Injury

Chapter 6

Iatrogenic Biliary Injury Surgical Management

Alex Zendel and Yaniv Fenig

Abstract

Bile duct injury (BDI) remains a critical complication following cholecystectomy. Prevention, early recognition, and appropriate management can significantly improve patient outcomes. In this chapter, we will discuss the current review of the surgical management of BDI, including prevention techniques during the cholecystectomy, intra-operative diagnosis of the injury, early evaluation and imaging, importance and challenges of the referrals to a hepatobiliary center, types and classification of biliary injuries, biliary drainage, and interventional procedures bridging to definitive repair, timing of surgical repair-early versus late, surgical repair techniques, evaluation and management of combined vasculo-biliary injury.

Keywords: prevention, intra-operative diagnosis, early referral, cholangiogram, percutaneous transhepatic biliary drainage, MRI/MRCP, early repair, delayed repair, hepato-jejunostomy, repair patency

1. Introduction

Laparoscopic cholecystectomy (LC) continues to be one of the most frequent surgical procedures performed in the US and the world, while bile duct injury (BDI) is the most morbid complication of LC [1]. Multiple preventive techniques reduced this complication rate [2], but BDI is still described in all LC's at 0.1–0.5% range [3]. Due to the high numbers of cholecystectomies performed, it is an enormous healthcare problem often leading to long-term physical and psychological morbidity to patients, with mortality described up to 7% [4]. It also is associated with multiple interventions and hospitalizations that generate a significant cost and burden to the patient and healthcare system [5].

Prevention of BDI is of paramount importance. Over the years, various classifications of biliary injuries have been proposed, and different methods have been described to prevent iatrogenic biliary tract lesions. The optimal treatment is influenced by the timing of recognition of the injury, the extent of BDI, the patient's clinical condition, and the availability of experienced hepatobiliary surgeons. This chapter aims to discuss the current updated management of iatrogenic BDI.

2. Safe cholecystectomy and prevention of BDI

2.1 Risk factors

Anatomical:

- Different variants of the cystic duct, such as short cystic duct, cystic duct running parallel to the common bile duct (CBD)
- Hepato-cystic duct
- Accessory cystic duct
- Aberrant bile ducts.

Patient-related:

- Acute or chronic inflammation
- Previous gastrointestinal or biliary surgery
- Obesity.

It has been demonstrated that the primary cause of BDI is the misinterpretation of biliary anatomy in 71–97% of all cases [6].

Over the years, various methods have been proposed and described to prevent iatrogenic biliary injury [7–9].

2.2 Surgical technique

2.2.1 Anatomical landmarks

- "Rouvière's sulcus"-2–5 cm sulcus running to the right of liver hilum, anterior to the caudate lobe, containing the right portal triad or right posterior branches, and usually easily visible during the laparoscopy. It can be considered a useful landmark site to start dissection of the hepato-cystic triangle during LC, and "no-pass" point to prevent the injury of the right hepatic artery [10].
- "Cystic lymph node" or Mascagni's node—always lies lateral to the biliary tree and should form the medial end point of dissection [11].
- "B-SAFE method"—by using five anatomic landmarks (B, bile duct; S, Rouvière's sulcis; A, hepatic artery; F, umbilical fissure; E, enteric/duodenum) to guide the dissection [12].
- The "line of safety" (**Figure 1**)—an imaginary line which extends from Rouviere's sulcus to the junction of the cystic and hilar plates, near the base of segment 4. It has been recently accepted as a relatively simple to define landmark representing the lower boundary for safe dissection [13].

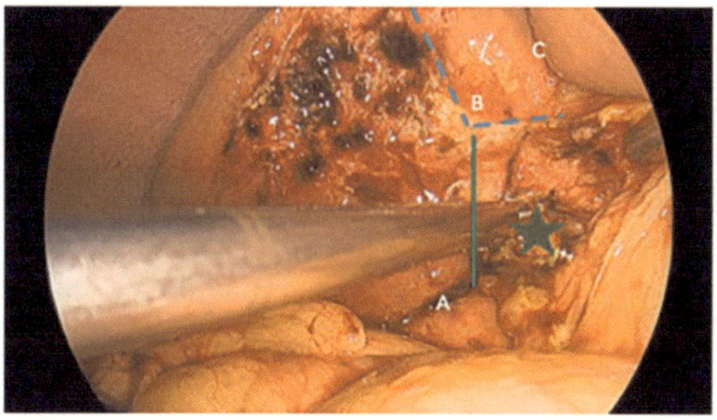

Figure 1.
Line of safety is an important intra-operative landmark to prevent BDI.

2.2.2 Dissection approach

- Infundibular method—dissection close to gallbladder infundibulum, still carries a risk of identifying dilated cystic duct as an infundibulum, while identifying CBD as a cystic duct [2]

- Fundus first/dome-down technique—a way of dissection from the gallbladder fundus up to the infundibulum away from Calot's triangle, so the gallbladder is left hanging on the cystic artery and cystic duct [14].

2.2.3 Final anatomical identification

The "critical view of safety (CVS)" technique (**Figure 2**) was introduced by Strasberg in 1995, and it is considered the gold standard to perform a safe cholecystectomy [9, 15]. It implies the identification of biliary structures during dissection and includes 3 criteria:

- The hepato-cystic triangle must be cleared of adipose and fibrotic tissues, and the CBD must not be exposed.

- The lower third of the gallbladder must be separated from the liver bed to expose the cystic plate.

- Two and only two structures should be seen entering the gallbladder.

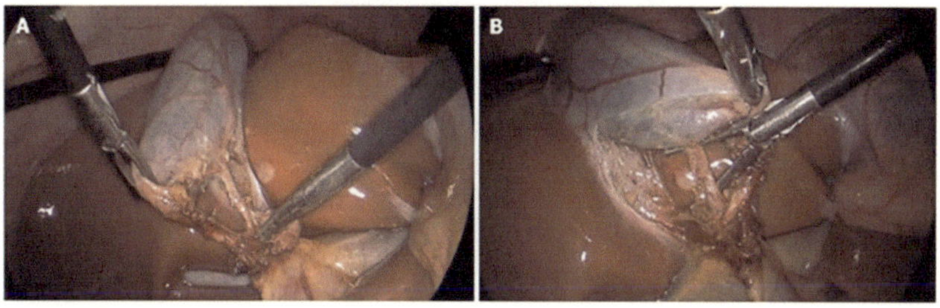

Figure 2.
Critical view of safety is a "gold standard" anatomical confirmation for safe cholecystectomy.

2.3 Intra-operative tools

2.3.1 Intra-operative cholangiography (IOC)

It has been proposed for the better declaration of biliary anatomy, detection of silent CBD stones, and reduction of incidence of BDIs [16]. The opinions about the "routine" or "selective" use of IOC still represent a matter of debate, but the selective approach is considered to have comparable chances of preventing and detecting BDI [17, 18]. However, it is highly advised to use IOC in any case of difficult LC or when there is a concern about biliary anatomy identification [18, 19].

2.3.2 Intra-operative ultrasound (IOUS)

It was shown to provide a highly sensitive mapping of the extra-hepatic biliary anatomy [20], but the difficult learning curve and the lack of randomized controlled trials have reduced its use in clinical practice.

2.3.3 Fluorescent cholangiography

It represents a novel intra-operative imaging technique that allows real-time enhanced visualization of the extrahepatic biliary tree by fluorescence, after the intravenous injection of the dye indocyanine green (ICG) [21]. It is a safe and useful method that became a common practice in difficult cholecystectomy [22, 23]. However, under the conditions of severe inflammation, this imaging can be less clear, and then, a strong consideration to bail out is suggested (**Figure 3**).

2.4 When to bail out

"Inflection point"—the moment the decision is made to complete formal laparoscopic cholecystectomy [24].

The general rule is that it should happen sooner than later before the injury happens. The consequences of bailing out are usually less morbid than those of biliary injury.

The following factors may influence personal surgeon's decision toward the inflection point [24, 25]:

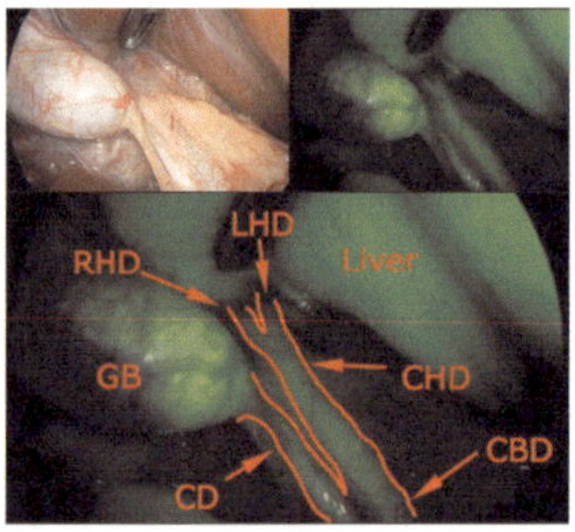

Figure 3.
A real-time enhanced visualization of the extrahepatic biliary tree by fluorescence, after the intravenous injection of the dye indocyanine green (ICG).

- Personal experience
- Inability to establish biliary anatomy
- Lack of intra-operative imaging modalities
- Time since the incision—60 minutes in general or 1.5 times the personal median time for LC completion
- Lack of colleague second opinion.

2.5 How to bail out

2.5.1 Laparoscopic subtotal or partial cholecystectomy

2.5.1.1 Fenestration type - preferred method

Fenestration of the gallbladder anterior wall, leaving the posterior wall attached to the liver, ablating the mucosa, and securing the cystic duct at its origin from the mucosal side within the gallbladder [26].

Pros: usually easy recognition of the cystic duct origin, reduced blood loss with no need to dissect the gallbladder bed from the liver, usually no need for a conversion to open procedure.

2.5.1.2 Reconstitution type - optional method: resection of most of the gallbladder and leaving the small stump

Pros: can prevent BDI in complex cases.

Cons: risk for neo-gallbladder appearance, recurrent stones, possible need for cholecystectomy completion, which is likely more complex and high-risk compared to the index one.

2.5.2 Conversion to the open procedure

Pros: usually allows cholecystectomy completion, improved recognition of the anatomy including vascular structures [24–26].

Cons: morbidity related to the open incision, lack of experience of modern surgeons in open cholecystectomy.

A general recommendation is that in all cases of complicated cholecystectomies, the surgeon must not hesitate when considering bailing out from the completion of formal LC, because the consequences may be dramatic.

3. Diagnosis

3.1 Clinical presentation

Depending on the timing of diagnosis and type of injury, it can be divided as followings by pathophysiology:

3.1.1 Asymptomatic/at the time of LC

3.1.1.1 Biliary leak

- The evolution of the symptoms is a function of bile accumulation based on the severity of the leak and is very subtle.
- Symptoms are usually non-specific (nausea, vomiting, bloating, widespread abdominal pain, general discomfort, and anorexia) till the development of bile peritonitis and sepsis.

3.1.1.2 Biliary obstruction and stricture

- It may have a different natural course based on the degree of obstruction (complete/partial) and location of the lesion (proximal/distal bile duct, main/lobar bile duct).
- Symptoms include obstructive jaundice and/or cholangitis, with abdominal pain, jaundice, and signs of infection/sepsis.

3.2 Non-invasive imaging

Radiologic investigations should be obtained for the correct identification of the damage, its extension, and gravity and to plan therapeutic strategies.

3.2.1 Ultrasonography (US)

A primary and easily available diagnostic tool that allows finding fluid collections, dilation of the bile ducts, and possibly associated vascular lesions, using Doppler evaluation [27].

3.2.2 Computed tomography (CT)

Superior to the US in detecting fluid collections, and guiding their percutaneous drainage, but similar to the US is not reliable in distinguishing bile leaks from other postoperative fluid collections, such as blood, pus, or serous fluid, because of their similar densities [28–30]. It can also show biliary obstruction with upstream dilatation, or long-term sequelae of a long-standing bile stricture, such as lobar hepatic atrophy or signs of secondary biliary cirrhosis. The CT scan is specifically useful to identify any associated vascular lesions.

3.2.3 Hepatobiliary scintigraphy (HS)

It seems to be more sensitive and specific than US or CT in detecting bile leaks and can provide functional information demonstrating the presence of an active leak [31]. However, its spatial resolution is poor, and the identification of the leak site can be challenging. In addition, it is limited in providing the exact anatomy of the whole biliary tree and in patients with hepatic dysfunction, and large leaks have poor sensitivity and can show no extrahepatic bile duct [32]. Because of those limitations, it is rarely used as a standalone test, and its use is replaced mostly by magnetic resonance imaging.

3.2.4 Magnetic resonance imaging with cholangiopancreatography (MRI/MRCP)

A non-invasive "gold standard" for the complete morphological evaluation of the biliary tree as it offers detailed information about the integrity of the biliary tract [28, 33]. The use of a gadolinium contrast agent during MRI/MRCP allows the detection of active bile leakage by direct visualization of contrast material extravasation into fluid collections in addition to demonstrating the anatomical site of the leakage and the type of BDI, and thus, it is superior to CT and US in specifying the collection as biloma [34, 35].

3.3 Invasive cholangiography

3.3.1 Types used

- Endoscopic retrograde cholangiopancreatography (ERCP) [32]
- Percutaneous transhepatic cholangiography (PTC)
- Intra-operative cholangiography (IOC).

3.3.2 General advantages

- A "gold standard" in identifying the presence of BDI and its type
- Provide exact biliary anatomy
- Allows the treatment of the injury by stenting and/or biliary drainage.

3.3.3 General disadvantages

- Nonnegligible risk of complications
- Lack of detection of extra biliary abnormality and surgical complications
- Non-visualization of the biliary tree upstream or downstream of the lesion—in case of complete transection or obstruction of the bile duct may require both ERCP and PTC to complete the biliary anatomy.

3.3.4 Specific considerations

3.3.4.1 ERCP

- Treatment of bile leak by papillotomy and pressure reduction and stenting [32, 36]
- In advanced injury as bridging till definitive repair in advanced

- In low-grade injury, usually with biliary opening less than 5 mm, as a definite treatment with no need for surgical repair
- Treatment of biliary obstruction by stenting
- Complications: pancreatitis, bleeding, and cholangitis.

3.3.4.2 PTC

- Usually requires dilation of the biliary tree, so easier to apply when some degree of biliary obstruction is present [37, 38]
- Treatment of bile leak by diversion of the bile flow
- When ERCP is not possible or not successful
- In the complete transection of the bile duct
- Treatment of biliary obstruction by diversion of the bile flow and stenting
- Recent experience showed satisfactory results with performing an extraluminal percutaneous endoscopic rendezvous procedure with stent placement to restore continuity of the bile duct [38, 39]. This procedure should be considered with caution, as it carries a risk for significant complications such as choledochoduodenal fistula [40].
- Complications: bleeding and cholangitis.

4. Classification

The location of BDI on the biliary tree is of primary importance in deciding management and predicting outcomes. We suggest using classification introduced by Strasberg in 1995 [7], as its comprehensive anatomical and functional injury description allows repair guidance and stratifies the risk for long-term complications, such as biliary stricture [41].

Figure 4 Strasberg classification.

Type A: bile leakage from either the minor bile ducts from gallbladder bed or the cystic duct.

Type B and C: occlusion (type B) or transection (type C) of aberrant right hepatic ducts.

Type D: lateral damage to the common bile duct resulting in a biliary leak.

Type E: involve the main ducts and are classified according to the level of injury in the biliary tree. Each type corresponds to the same type of Bismuth classification:

E1 - >2 cm from the confluence.

E2 - <2 cm from the confluence.

E3 - in the hilum, right and left duct are not separated.

E4 - in the hilum, right and left duct are separated.

E5 - in the hilum, combined with type C.

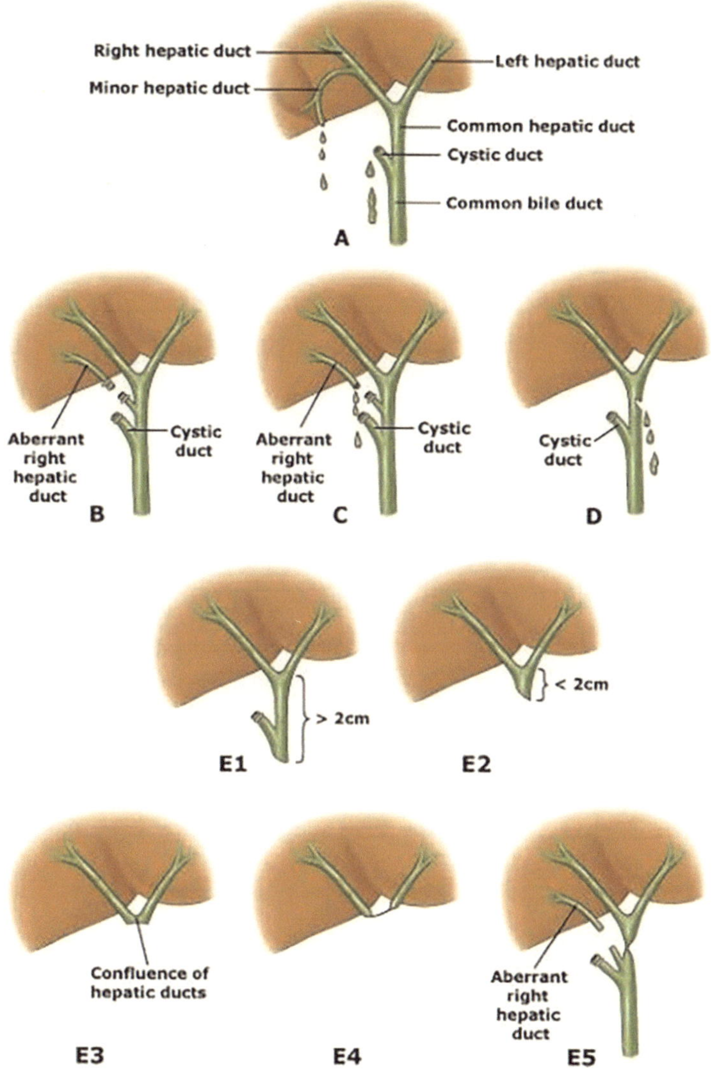

Figure 4.
Strasberg's classification of BDI.

5. Timing of diagnosis and repair

Early and delayed repair are both acceptable approaches to a definite repair of BDI. The big question exists regarding an exact definition of "early" vs. "delayed". The data is mixed, and the time from the initial surgery is defined as between 0 and 21 days for early [5, 8, 12, 13] and after 4–6 weeks as "delayed" [8, 12].

Advantages of early approach:

- Reduced inflammation—if done early enough
- Decreased morbidity of temporary biliary drainage

- Decreased psychological trauma to the patient
- Faster recovery and a quicker return to the regular lifestyle.

Advantages of delayed approach:

- More detailed diagnosis of the degree and type of BDI
- Reduction in inflammation
- Improved anatomic visualization
- Delay allows undiagnosed associated vascular injuries to be identified.
- Provides the surgeon a better roadmap for developing an operative plan for definitive reconstruction.

5.1 Choice of the early versus delayed repair

5.1.1 Timing

Based on most recent evidence, we recommend considering early repair within 48–72 hours from the injury [40, 42, 43]. Some data suggests the earlier the repair, the better the results [4, 44, 45] whereas other support comparable good outcomes within 72 hours timeframe [46].

When missed the opportunity window of 48–72 hours for an early repair, it is advised to delay it for at least 4–6 weeks [37, 43, 47]. This will allow to decrease the degree of local inflammation, control infection, and optimize the conditions for a complex reconstruction.

5.1.2 Expertise

The repair of a bile duct injury is a complicated procedure, and there is clear evidence that the best results are obtained at a center with experienced hepatobiliary surgeons [43, 48–50]. It is a single most important factor in the success of the repair. At attempt to perform an immediate repair by an unexperienced surgeon is associated with worse outcomes and can compromise the future repair by a specialist, in case of repair complications [43, 50].

5.1.3 Type of injury

In the presence or suspicion for a vascular injury, one should consider delaying a repair to complete a comprehensive work-up and to allow the injury present and establish its clinical significance [43, 51].

5.2 Early repair

5.2.1 Immediate recognition of the injury at the time of LC

After the prevention of the injury, the surgeon's awareness to suspect and evaluate for a BDI is the second most important factor in determining the patient prognosis.

5.2.1.1 Immediate intra-operative repair

If the required surgical expertise is present, we suggest following steps:

1. Conversion to an open procedure
2. Careful surgical exploration and identification of important structures and the injury
3. Confirmation of injury type with intra-operative cholangiography
4. The preference is to image both proximal and distal direction of the biliary tree if possible.
5. Consider IOUS if vascular injury is suspected [51]
6. Immediate repair according to the type of injury.

5.2.1.2 Early transfer to a tertiary referral center

If the competent surgeon capable of performing a biliary reconstruction is not present, we advise to follow the next steps:

1. DO NOT convert to an open procedure. This may expose the patient to an additional morbidity and make the definite repair more complicated [43, 48, 50]. The acceptable reason to convert may be bleeding difficult to control laparoscopically.
2. If possible, evaluate the injury type by intra-operative cholangiogram.
3. Place a drain [52].
4. Transfer a patient as soon as possible to a tertiary hepatobiliary referral center—that provides better outcomes that immediate repair by less experienced surgeon.
5. Provide as much relevant information as possible with the referral. Additional imaging, such as MRI/MRCP, can be performed while waiting for a transfer.

5.2.2 Early recognition after completion of cholecystectomy

At the same admission it presents as described earlier symptoms and signs of biliary leak, obstruction, or both. A general recommendation is that any alteration in the normal postoperative course after LC must suggest a possible damage to the biliary tract. Sometimes, the evolution of biliary symptoms is subtle, so high degree of clinical suspicion and careful clinical evaluation of patients are essential. It will allow the thorough and prompt inpatient evaluation and/or referral to a tertiary specialty center.

The diagnosis after the discharge is often made based on clinical symptoms, which means more advanced and complicated problem, or based on abnormal lab tests, in case of milder injury.

To allow the chance of early repair, one should apply similar principles as described in case of intra-operative injury recognition:

5.2.2.1 Perform prompt biliary imaging to evaluate the type of the injury and provide the drainage of biliary system

US:

- Initial imaging
- Identification of biliary dilatation, fluid collections, and vascular injuries by Doppler.

MRCP:

- First-line non-invasive imaging.
- Can be confirmatory for the type of injury.

CT:

- Important to rule out associated vascular injury
- Allows imaging-guided percutaneous drainage of the collections.

ERCP:

- First-line confirmatory biliary imaging.
- Allows drainage and stenting.
- In mild grade injuries (A-D) can be sufficient as the only treatment with no need for operative intervention.

PTC:

- First-line procedure for drainage and stenting when MRI/MRCP confirms complete transection or obstruction of the bile ducts
- Usually needed in type E injuries is temporary bridging treatment till the delayed repair [40]
- Second-line procedure for drainage and stenting if ERCP not feasible.

Drain any biloma or abscess percutaneously if operative drain is not present or is not providing adequate drainage—to prevent and treat bile peritonitis and sepsis, as well as to control the ongoing leak [52].

5.2.2.2 Make the decision about the possibility of early repair, based on factors discussed earlier

- Presence of competent hepatobiliary surgeon

- Timing of the diagnosis—up to 72 hours from the injury
- Absence of vascular injury.

5.3 Delayed repair

5.3.1 The conditions leading to choosing the delayed repair approach

- Late recognition—beyond 72 hours from the injury
- Need for a comprehensive work-up to determine the type and degree of the injury
- Delays in transfer to a referral hepatobiliary center, related to geographic distance, transportation resources, and bed availability [40, 53]
- Patient hemodynamic instability or uncontrolled sepsis [52]
- Patient complex medical background requiring pre-operative optimization [40].

6. Management and repair of minor BDI—types A-D

6.1 Type A injury

6.1.1 Non-operative management

- Draining an abdominal collection and controlling a leak alone may be a sufficient treatment [49, 52, 54]
- If the leak is not controlled by a drainage alone, proceed with ERCP, which success in the minor BDI with low output leaks is between 87% and 100% [49, 55–60].

6.1.2 Operative repair

- The operative intervention reserved for minority of the cases, where the leak is not resolving after ERCP and drainage or when discovered intra-operatively
- Technique—surgical ligation of a cystic duct stump or oversewing an accessory duct at the gallbladder bed provides simple and reliable solution.

6.2 Type B injury

6.2.1 Non-operative management

- Is appropriate when a segmental or accessory ligated duct is small (usually up to 3 mm) and cholangiography demonstrates adequate drainage of the segment with an injured bile duct.

- Temporary percutaneous drainage (PTC) can be placed to control cholangitis in the obstructed segment.

6.2.2 Operative repair

- Is warranted if the injured duct is bigger (more than 3 mm), drain multiple hepatic segments, no adequate drainage is confirmed by cholangiography or if there is recurrent cholangitis is present despite maximal percutaneous drainage

- Reconstruction of injured duct by Roux n Y Hepato-Jejunostomy—when duct is bigger, and reconstruction is technically feasible

- Hepatic resection of the obstructed segment to control recurrent cholangitis—when reconstruction is not feasible.

6.3 Type C injury

6.3.1 Non-operative management

- Is appropriate when segmental or accessory leaking duct is small (up to 2–3 mm), cholangiography demonstrates adequate drainage of the segment with an injured bile duct.

- Temporary endoscopic or percutaneous drainage may be required to control the leak.

6.3.2 Operative repair

- Ligation of injured duct—when the duct is small and adequate segmental drainage confirmed by cholangiography, but the leak is not controlled.

- Reconstruction of injured duct by Roux n Y Hepato-Jejunostomy—when the duct is large, and no adequate drainage is confirmed by cholangiography.

Injuries grade D and above usually will require operative intervention.

6.4 Type D injury

6.4.1 Non-operative management

- ERCP with papillotomy and possible stenting can be appropriate when the side injury of the bile duct is small, usually less than 5 mm, and the leak is low output [49, 56].

- Can be attempted on the high-output leaks as well, but the chance for success with endoscopic treatment only is low [54]

- In addition, an abdominal drain for controlling the leak should be placed [49, 54].

6.4.2 Operative repair

- Is recommended if recognized intra-operatively, after the failure of endoscopic treatment or large injury and leak are demonstrated on the imaging [49, 56–58]
- Usually, the choledochotomy can be repaired primarily with 5–0 or 6–0 absorbable sutures.
- In case of very large side injury, debridement of the duct may be required and primary duct-to-duct anastomosis with healthy duct edges performed [45, 60].
- Consider surgical or endoscopic stenting in addition to the surgical repair [45, 61, 62].

7. Management and repair of major BDI—types E injury (transection, clipping, or stricture of major bile ducts)

7.1 Non-operative management

7.1.1 ERCP

- Rarely can be successful as a standalone management without surgical reconstruction and is associated with high morbidity [54, 63]
- Consider as an alternative for surgical reconstruction in patients with very-high perioperative risk due to medical co-morbidities and surgical history [40]
- Can be attempted when there is at least partially documented MRCP confirmed of the bile duct, or a very close proximity of the proximal and distal biliary stumps two biliary stumps [64]
- This should be performed only by highly experienced biliary endoscopist, as it might carry the risk for significant morbidity endoscopists [40, 60, 63, 64].
- Although less investigated in the literature, long-term (at 10 years) outcomes of endoscopic treatment with stent placement appeared to be good and effective in patients with postoperative biliary strictures [65–67].

7.1.2 PTC

- A necessary and effective bridging biliary procedure while waiting for a delayed repair [40, 67, 68]
- Specifically successful in cases of complete obstruction of the bile duct, or when a significant stricture present, and ERCP is not successful or feasible [67, 68]
- PTC in the presence of bile leakage may be more difficult because of non-dilated bile ducts but still leads to a technical success of 90% and a short-term clinical success of 70–80% in expertise centers [67–69].

7.2 Primary anastomosis of the bile duct-choledocholedochostomy

7.2.1 Why to attempt-advantages on bilioenteric reconstruction

- Less technically complex
- Shorter operative time-important in case the patient is septic or unstable.
- Less short-term post-operative complications [70].
- Allows favorable access for endoscopic treatment of anastomotic complications.

7.2.2 Can be performed in selected cases-conditions to perform

- If there is no significant loss of bile duct tissue (usually less than 1 cm)
- Proximal and distal biliary stump ends can be opposed without tension.
- Recommended in settings of early reconstruction only, usually not feasible in a delayed fashion, as the chronic inflammation and fibrosis interferes with an ability to perform tension free repair [57, 71]
- When no vascular injury is present

7.2.3 An exceptional clinical judgment is required to decide about the primary bile duct

reconstruction as this approach is associated with increased failure rate compared to bilioenteric reconstruction, especially when it is performed beyond the conditions mentioned above [50, 57, 72].

7.2.4 Choledocholedochostomy-operative technique

- Debridement of bile duct ends, till getting satisfactory healthy tissue
- Extended Kocher maneuver can help with mobilization of a distal bile duct and allow approximation of both ends
- Consider placement of biliary stent or T-tube
- Performing an end-to-end fashion anastomosis with absorbable sutures.
- Drain placement.

7.3 Bilioenteric reconstruction—Roux-en-Y hepatojejunostomy

It represents a gold standard surgical repair of major bile duct injuries and is being performed as a definite repair in most cases of BDI [7, 43, 49, 73]

7.3.1 Advantages

- Allows resection of the bile duct and performing high biliary anastomosis
- It which carries better blood supply by communicating vessels from peribiliary plexus at the level of biliary bifurcation, which usually remain intact even after high grade BDI
- Allows tension-free anastomosis
- Overall, less anastomotic complication and reduced need for reoperation than the primary bile duct repair [50, 57, 72–74].

7.3.2 Roux-en-Y Hepato-jejunostomy-surgical technique

- Closure of the distal bile duct stump
- Proximal small bowel Roux limb creation
- Placement of biliary stent through the anastomosis
- End-to-side or side-to-side proximal bile duct-to-bowel anastomosis with absorbable sutures
- Creation of Y limb and jejunojejunostomy (**Figure** 5).

7.3.3 The details of repair vary depending upon the grade of the injury

7.3.3.1 Type E1–2

Single duct bilioenteric anastomosis.

7.3.3.2 Type E3

- If the bile duct bifurcation maintained as a single orifice allowing technically feasible reconstruction—can perform single bilioenteric anastomosis

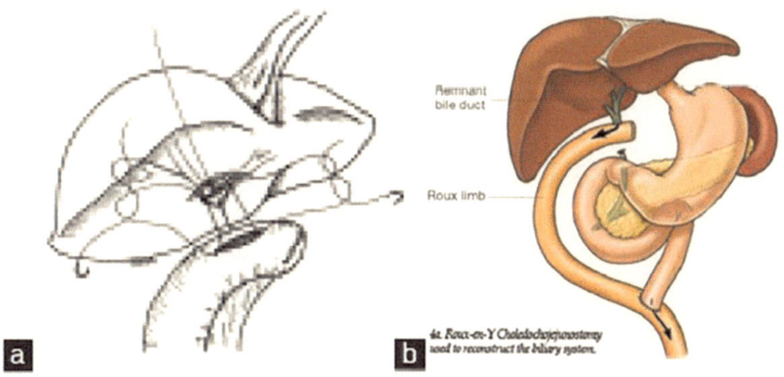

Figure 5.
Roux-en-Y Hepato-jejunostomy - surgical technique.

- If not, two separate right and left anastomoses should be performed.

7.3.3.3 Type E4

- Two separate right and left biliary enteric anastomoses are usually required.
- As an alternative both biliary branches can be reconstructed together as a single orifice.
- In rare cases, suitable duct length outside the hepatic parenchyma cannot be obtained, these cases necessitate isolation of the intrahepatic biliary system, and IOUS may be necessary in these situations.

7.3.3.4 Type E5

- Principles of E4 type are applied.
- The additional duct may be ligated or reconstructed based on the principles for segmental accessory duct injury management, described earlier.

7.3.3.5 Technical solutions in complicated cases

- In order to achieve sufficient bile duct caliber side-to-side technique may be preferred, including opening the left hepatic duct but keeping the posterior wall of the bifurcation to preserve the blood supply, according to the Hepp-Couinaud technique [75, 76].

8. Vasculobiliary injury (VBI)

This is defined as a combined injury to a bile duct and to an accompanying major blood vessels in the porta hepatis.

Types of VBI [75]:

- Classic (over 90% of VBI)—Right hepatic artery (RHA) injury
- Extreme (less than 10% of VBI)—Combined RHA and main or right portal vein (PV) injury.

8.1 Classic VBI

8.1.1 Injury to the RHA below the biliary confluence (usually type E1/E2)

Does not usually cause a clinically significant ischemic injury to the liver parenchyma, due to a shunt that occurs immediately from the left hepatic artery (LHA) traveling via the transverse hilar marginal artery (THMA) to the right liver [76].

8.1.2 Injury to the RHA above the biliary confluence of the ducts

- Will disrupt the collateral biliary blood supply including THMA.

- Possible clinical presentations include development of small areas of right hepatic lobe ischemia with possible subsequent abscesses formation.
- Chronic atrophy of the right hepatic lobe, which is usually clinically unsignificant due to intact portal blood supply.

8.2 Impact of VBI on definite repair approach

8.2.1 Diagnosis

- US with Doppler can provide some information.
- CT scan with IV contrast usually required as a part of work-up for high-grade biliary injury (types E) to rule out.
- High level of suspicion for VBI, based on high grade biliary injury or intra-operative bleeding will mandate the imaging work-up, making the immediate repair unlikely.

8.2.2 Timing of repair

- VBI increases the risk for repair stenosis repair should not be neglected as it will lead to extensive morbidity and the need for endoscopic or percutaneous interventions [75].
- In severe and untreated cases, it can lead to late biliary cirrhosis with portal hypertension.
- To avoid this the repair should be delayed for several weeks to allow the ischemic injury to delineate and ensure the anastomosis is done to well vascularized tissue.

8.2.3 Surgical approach to repair

- Avoid primary duct to duct anastomosis [71, 75].
- Hepaticojejunostomy is the repair of choice.
- A resection of extrahepatic bile duct and the anastomosis at the level of bifurcation is preferred—to achieve adequately perfused margins.
- While lowering the hilar plate to achieve sufficient proximal biliary stump, care should be taken to avoid additional devascularization of peribiliary vascular plexus.
- Described above side-to-side hepato-jejunostomy technique can provide a solution for creation of wide and well-vascularized anastomosis.

8.2.4 Arterial reconstruction

- Usually, it is not possible to reconstruct the RHA and indeed it is not necessary, because of little clinical significance of liver disfunction.

8.2.5 Outcomes

- With the right surgical classic VBI can be managed with the outcomes comparable to BDI without vascular injury [40].

8.3 Extreme VBI

- Rare and devastating injury
- Can be associated with "dome-down" approach to a shrunken gallbladder which results in massive bleeding from both the portal vein and hepatic artery [77].
- The main priority—bleeding control
- As opposed to arterial injury, the likelihood of hepatic ischemia is high in PV injury.
- It can require right hepatectomy in case of RPV injury or PV reconstruction and even liver transplantation in case of main PV injury.
- In this scenario, the short- and long-term outcomes are dismal with up to 60% mortality risk [78].

9. Conclusions

- Bile duct injury (BDI) remains a critical complication following cholecystectomy.
- Early recognition and appropriate management can significantly improve patient outcomes.
- Prevention of biliary injury during cholecystectomy is of paramount importance and includes recognition of anatomical landmarks and a critical view of safety achievement, precise surgical technique, use of intra-operative imaging, and timely bailing out from a completion of a standard laparoscopic cholecystectomy.
- Diagnosis of biliary injury is made based on clinical picture of biliary leak or obstruction, ultrasonography, cross-sectional imaging, and cholangiography.
- Strasberg classification of BDI is the most comprehensive to define the type and extent of the injury and guide the surgical repair.
- Early and delayed repair are both acceptable approaches to a definite repair of BDI. We recommend choosing an early repair up to 72 hours from the injury and if missed this opportunity, to delay it for at least 4 weeks.

- The BDI repair should be performed by an experienced Hepato-Pancreato-Biliary surgeon, and thus, the presence of such an expertise is the most important factor in deciding the timing of the repair.
- If needed, early and organized referral to a tertiary center is the first time limiting critical step of BDI management.
- Intraoperative recognition of the injury allows the best chance for an early repair and can prevent the morbidity associated with a delayed repair.
- Prior to a decision for the repair, the complete understanding of biliary anatomy and injury type is required and can be achieved by MRI/MRCP, ERCP or PTC.
- The latter two are also important for a temporary control of biliary injury.
- PTC is particularly useful as a bridging treatment for high-grade injuries with a loss of biliary continuity while waiting for a delayed repair.
- As a part of surgical management, the intra-abdominal biliary sepsis and leak should be controlled with appropriate drainage.
- The definite surgical management of low-grade Strasberg types A-D injuries can include biliary drainage only, primary repair of the bile duct or duct-to-duct biliary reconstruction.
- In cases of significant bile duct tissue loss and tension associated with primary repair, bilioenteric reconstruction with Roux-en-Y hepato-jejunostomy is recommended.
- High-grade Strasberg type E injuries should be always repaired with Roux-en-Y hepatojejunostomy.
- The proper surgical technique allowing reconstruction of healthy and well-vascularized bile duct is an absolute condition for a success and long-term patency of the repair, so the resection of the extrahepatic bile duct and high anastomosis at the level of biliary bifurcation is always preferred.
- Associate vascular injury defined as vasculobiliary injury (VBI) should be always ruled out in BDI evaluation.
- Most common is right hepatic artery injury and it mandates delaying the definite surgical repair to allow the ischemic injury to delineate and ensure the anastomosis is done to well-vascularized tissue.
- With appropriate management, comparable outcomes to BDI without vascular injury can be achieved.
- Rare and devastating portal vein injuries often require partial liver resections and are associated with high morbidity and mortality.

Acknowledgements

Chirag S Desai, MD, University of North Carolina at Chapel Hill, Division of Abdominal Transplantation for the mentorship, guidance, and friendship.

Thanks

Thanks to my family, colleagues, and mentors, this book chapter publishing would not be possible without their support.

Author details

Alex Zendel[1*] and Yaniv Fenig[2]

1 University of North Carolina at Chapel Hill, NC, US

2 SUNY Downstate Health Sciences University, Brooklyn, NY, US

*Address all correspondence to: drazendel@gmail.com

References

[1] Ingraham AM, Cohen ME, Ko CY, Hall BL. A current profile and assessment of north American cholecystectomy: Results from the American college of surgeons national surgical quality improvement program. Journal of the American College of Surgeons. 2010;**211**:176-186

[2] Daly SC, Deziel DJ, Li X, et al. Current practices in biliary surgery: Do we practice what we teach? Surgical Endoscopy. 2016;**30**:3345-3350

[3] Stilling NM, Fristrup C, Wettergren A, et al. Long-term outcome after early repair of iatrogenic bile duct injury. A national Danish multicentre study. HPB. 2015;**17**:394-400

[4] Pekolj J, Alvarez FA, Palavecino M, Sa'nchez Claria R, Mazza O, de Santibañes E. Intraoperative management and repair of bile duct injuries sustained during 10,123 laparoscopic cholecystectomies in a high-volume Re- ferral Center. Journal of the American College of Surgeons. 2013;**216**:894-901

[5] Booij KAC, de Reuver PR, van Dieren S, et al. Long-term impact of bile duct injury on morbidity, mortality, quality of life, and work related limitations. Annals of Surgery. Jul 2018; **268**(1):143-150

[6] Nuzzo G, Giuliante F, Giovannini I, Ardito F, D'Acapito F, Vellone M, et al. Bile duct injury during laparoscopic cholecystectomy: Results of an Italian national survey on 56 591 cholecystectomies. Archives of Surgery. 2005;**140**(10):986-992. DOI: 10.1001/archsurg.140.10.986

[7] Strasberg SM, Hertl M, Soper NJ. An analysis of the problem of biliary injury during laparoscopic cholecystectomy. Journal of the American College of Surgeons. 1995;**180**(1):101-125

[8] Pesce A, Palmucci S, La Greca G, Puleo S. Iatrogenic bile duct injury: Impact and management challenges. Clinical and Experimental Gastroenterology. 2019;**12**:121-128. DOI: 10.2147/CEG.S169492

[9] Strasberg Steven M, Michael BL. The critical view of safety: Why it is not the only method of ductal identification within the standard of care in laparoscopic cholecystectomy. Annals of Surgery. 2017;**265**(3):464-465. DOI: 10.1097/SLA.0000000000002054

[10] Hugh TB, Kelly MD, Mekisic A. Rouvière's sulcus: A useful landmark in laparoscopic cholecystectomy. The British Journal of Surgery. 1997;**84**(9): 1253-1254. DOI: 10.1046/j.1365-2168.1997.02769.x

[11] Ferzli G, Timoney M, Nazir S, Swedler D, Fingerhut A. Importance of the node of calot in gallbladder neck dissection: An important landmark in the standardized approach to the laparoscopic cholecystectomy. Journal of Laparoendoscopic & Advanced Surgical Techniques. Part A. 2015;**25**(1):28-32. DOI: 10.1089/lap.2014.0195

[12] Sutherland F, Dixon E. The importance of cognitive map placement in bile duct injuries. Canadian Journal of Surgery. 2017;**60**(6):424-425. DOI: 10.1503/cjs.008816

[13] Greene B, Tsang M, Jayaraman S. The inferior boundary of dissection as a novel landmark for safe laparoscopic cholecystectomy. HPB: The Official Journal of the International Hepato

Pancreato Biliary Association. 2021; **23**(7):981-983. DOI: 10.1016/j.hpb.2021.02.004

[14] Neri V, Ambrosi A, Fersini A, Tartaglia N, Valentino TP. Antegrade dissection in laparoscopic cholecystectomy. Journal of the Society of Laparoscopic Surgeons. 2007;**11**(2):225-228

[15] Strasberg SM, Brunt LM. Rationale and use of the critical view of safety in laparoscopic cholecystectomy. Journal of the American College of Surgeons. 2010; **211**(1):132-138. DOI: 10.1016/j.jamcollsurg.2010.02.053

[16] Pesce A, Portale TR, Minutolo V, Scilletta R, Li Destri G, Puleo S. Bile duct injury during laparoscopic cholecystectomy without intraoperative cholangiography: A retrospective study on 1100 selected patients. Digestive Surgery. 2012;**29**(4):310-314. DOI: 10.1159/000341660

[17] Sajid MS, Leaver C, Haider Z, Worthington T, Karanjia N, Singh KK. Routine on-table cholangiography during cholecystectomy: A systematic review. Annals of the Royal College of Surgeons of England. 2012;**94**(6): 375-380. DOI: 10.1308/003588412X13373405385331

[18] Törnqvist B, Strömberg C, Akre O, Enochsson L, Nilsson M. Selective intraoperative cholangiography and risk of bile duct injury during cholecystectomy. The British Journal of Surgery. 2015;**102**(8):952-958. DOI: 10.1002/bjs.9832

[19] Törnqvist B, Waage A, Zheng Z, Ye W, Nilsson M. Severity of acute cholecystitis and risk of iatrogenic bile duct injury during cholecystectomy, a population-based case-control study. World Journal of Surgery. 2016;**40**(5): 1060-1067. DOI: 10.1007/s00268-015-3365-1

[20] Dili A, Bertrand C. Laparoscopic ultrasonography as an alternative to intraoperative cholangiography during laparoscopic cholecystectomy. World Journal of Gastroenterology. 2017; **23**(29):5438-5450. DOI: 10.3748/wjg.v23.i29.5438

[21] Ishizawa T, Bandai Y, Kokudo N. Fluorescent cholangiography using indocyanine green for laparoscopic cholecystectomy: An initial experience. Archives of Surgery. 2009;**144**(4): 381-382. DOI: 10.1001/archsurg.2009.9

[22] Pesce A, Piccolo G, La Greca G, Puleo S. Utility of fluorescent cholangiography during laparoscopic cholecystectomy: A systematic review. World Journal of Gastroenterology. 2015;**21**(25):7877-7883. DOI: 10.3748/wjg.v21.i25.7877

[23] Calabro KA, Harmon CM, Vali K. Fluorescent cholangiography in laparoscopic cholecystectomy and the use in Pediatric patients. Journal of Laparoendoscopic & Advanced Surgical Techniques. Part A. 2020;**30**(5):586-589. DOI: 10.1089/lap.2019.0204

[24] Strasberg SM. A three-step conceptual roadmap for avoiding bile duct injury in laparoscopic cholecystectomy: An invited perspective review. Journal of Hepato-Biliary-Pancreatic Sciences. 2019;**26**(4):123-127. DOI: 10.1002/jhbp.616

[25] Bourgouin S, Mancini J, Monchal T, Calvary R, Bordes J, Balandraud P. How to predict difficult laparoscopic cholecystectomy? Proposal for a simple preoperative scoring system. American Journal of Surgery. 2016;**212**(5):873-881. DOI: 10.1016/j.amjsurg.2016.04.003

[26] Bornman PC, Terblanche J. Subtotal cholecystectomy: For the difficult gallbladder in portal hypertension and cholecystitis. Surgery. 1985;**98**(1):1-6

[27] Wigham A, Alexander GL. Radiologic assessment of hepatobiliary surgical complications. Seminars in Ultrasound, CT, and MR. 2013; **34**(1):18-31. DOI: 10.1053/j.sult.2012.11.002

[28] Jabłońska B, Lampe P. Iatrogenic bile duct injuries: Etiology, diagnosis and management. World Journal of Gastroenterology. 2009;**15**(33): 4097-4104. DOI: 10.3748/wjg.15.4097

[29] Mulé S, Colosio A, Cazejust J, Kianmanesh R, Soyer P, Hoeffel C. Imaging of the postoperative liver: Review of normal appearances and common complications. Abdominal Imaging. 2015;**40**(7):2761-2776. DOI: 10.1007/s00261-015-0459-z

[30] Lee CM, Stewart L, Way LW. Postcholecystectomy abdominal bile collections. Archives of Surgery. 2000; **135**(5):538-542. DOI: 10.1001/archsurg.135.5.538

[31] Tripathi M, Chandrashekar N, Kumar R, Thomas EJ, Agarwal S, Bal CS, et al. Hepatobiliary scintigraphy. An effective tool in the management of bile leak following laparoscopic cholecystectomy. Clinical Imaging. 2004;**28**(1):40-43. DOI: 10.1016/S0899-7071(03)00035-4

[32] Barkun AN, Rezieg M, Mehta SN, Pavone E, Landry S, Barkun JS, et al. Postcholecystectomy biliary leaks in the laparoscopic era: Risk factors, presentation, and management. McGill Gallstone Treatment Group. Gastrointestinal Endoscopy. 1997;**45**(3): 277-282. DOI: 10.1016/s0016-5107(97)70270-0

[33] Reddy S, Lopes Vendrami C, Mittal P, Borhani AA, Moreno CC, Miller FH. MRI evaluation of bile duct injuries and other post-cholecystectomy complications. Abdominal Radiology (NY). 2021;**46**(7):3086-3104. DOI: 10.1007/s00261-020-02947-z

[34] Palmucci S, Mauro LA, La Scola S, Incarbone S, Bonanno G, Milone P, et al. Magnetic resonance cholangiopancreatography and contrast-enhanced magnetic resonance cholangiopancreatography versus endoscopic ultrasonography in the diagnosis of extrahepatic biliary pathology. La Radiologia Medica. 2010; **115**(5):732-746. DOI: 10.1007/s11547-010-0526-z

[35] Aduna M, Larena JA, Martín D, Martínez-Guereñu B, Aguirre I, Astigarraga E. Bile duct leaks after laparoscopic cholecystectomy: Value of contrast-enhanced MRCP. Abdominal Imaging. 2005;**30**(4):480-487. DOI: 10.1007/s00261-004-0276-2

[36] Rainio M, Lindström O, Udd M, Haapamäki C, Nordin A, Kylänpää L. Endoscopic therapy of biliary injury after cholecystectomy. Digestive Diseases and Sciences. 2018;**63**(2): 474-480. DOI: 10.1007/s10620-017-4768-7

[37] Fidelman N, Kerlan RK Jr, Laberge JM, Gordon RL. Accuracy of percutaneous transhepatic cholangiography in predicting the location and nature of major bile duct injuries. Journal of Vascular and Interventional Radiology. 2011;**22**(6): 884-892. DOI: 10.1016/j.jvir.2011.02.007

[38] Schreuder AM, Booij KAC, de Reuver PR, van Delden OM, van Lienden KP, Besselink MG, et al. Percutaneous-endoscopic rendezvous procedure for the management of bile

duct injuries after cholecystectomy: Short- and long-term outcomes. Endoscopy. 2018;**50**(6):577-587. DOI: 10.1055/s-0043-123935

[39] Lindemann J, Kloppers C, Burmeister S, Bernon M, Jonas E. Mind the gap! Extraluminal percutaneous-endoscopic rendezvous with a self-expanding metal stent for restoring continuity in major bile duct injury: A case series. International Journal of Surgery Case Reports. 2019;**60**:340-344. DOI: 10.1016/j.ijscr.2019.06.059

[40] Zendel A, Kumar A, Serrano P, de Oliveira GC, Button J, Gebre B, et al. Management of major injuries to the bile duct at a hepatobiliary specialty referral center. The American Surgeon. 16 Feb 2022:31348211063553. DOI: 10.1177/00031348211063553. PMID: 35172613. [Epub ahead of print]

[41] Walsh RM, Henderson JM, Vogt DP, Brown N. Long-term outcome of biliary reconstruction for bile duct injuries from laparoscopic cholecystectomies. Surgery. 2007;**142**(4):450-456. DOI: 10.1016/j.surg.2007.07.008

[42] Stewart L. Iatrogenic biliary injuries: Identification, classification, and management. Surgical Clinics. 2014; **94**(2):297-310

[43] Wang X, Yu WL, Fu XH, Zhu B, Zhao T, Zhang YJ. Early versus delayed surgical repair and referral for patients with bile duct injury: A systematic review and meta-analysis. Annals of Surgery. 2020;**271**(3):449-459

[44] Rystedt J, Lindell G, Montgomery A. Bile duct injuries associated with 55,134 cholecystectomies: Treatment and outcome from a National Perspective. World Journal of Surgery. 2016; **40**(1):73-80. DOI: 10.1007/s00268-015-3281-4

[45] Silva MA, Coldham C, Mayer AD, Bramhall SR, Buckels JA, Mirza DF. Specialist outreach service for on-table repair of iatrogenic bile duct injuries - A new kind of 'travelling surgeon'. Annals of the Royal College of Surgeons of England. 2008;**90**(3):243-246. DOI: 10.1308/003588408X261663

[46] Dominguez-Rosado I, Sanford DE, Liu J, Hawkins WG, Mercado MA. Timing of surgical repair after bile duct injury impacts postoperative complications but not Anas - Tomotic patency. Annals of Surgery. 2016; **264**(3):544-553

[47] Lillemoe KD, Melton GB, Cameron JL, Pitt HA, Campbell KA, Talamini MA, et al. Postoperative bile duct strictures: Management and outcome in the 1990s. Annals of Surgery. 2000 Sep;**232**(3):430-441. DOI: 10.1097/00000658-200009000-00015

[48] Strasberg SM. Biliary injury in laparoscopic surgery: Part 2. Changing the culture of cholecystectomy. Journal of the American College of Surgeons. 2005;**201**(4):604-611. DOI: 10.1016/j.jamcollsurg.2005.04.032

[49] Perera MT, Silva MA, Hegab B, Muralidharan V, Bramhall SR, Mayer AD, et al. Specialist early and immediate repair of post-laparoscopic cholecystectomy bile duct injuries is associated with an improved long-term outcome. Annals of Surgery. 2011; **253**(3):553-560. DOI: 10.1097/SLA.0b013e318208fad3

[50] Stewart L, Way LW. Bile duct injuries during laparoscopic cholecystectomy. Factors that influence the results of treatment. Archives of Surgery. 1995 Oct;**130**(10):1123-1128. DOI: 10.1001/archsurg.1995.01430100101019

[51] Alves A, Farges O, Nicolet J, Watrin T, Sauvanet A, Belghiti J. Incidence and consequence of an hepatic artery injury in patients with postcholecystectomy bile duct strictures. Annals of Surgery. 2003;**238**(1): 93-96. DOI: 10.1097/01.sla.0000074983.39297.c5

[52] Krige JE, Bornman PC, Kahn D. Bile leaks and sepsis: Drain now, fix later. Archives of Surgery. 2010;**145**(8):763. DOI: 10.1001/archsurg.2010.154

[53] Ray S, Sanyal S, Das S, Jana K, Das AK, Khamrui S. Outcomes of surgery for post-cholecystectomy bile duct injuries: An audit from a tertiary referral center. Journal of Visceral Surgery. 2020;**157**(1):3-11. DOI: 10.1016/j.jviscsurg.2019.08.005

[54] Kimura T, Suzuki K, Umehara Y, Kawabe A, Wada H. Features and management of bile leaks after laparoscopic cholecystectomy. Journal of Hepato-Biliary-Pancreatic Surgery. 2005;**12**(1):61-64. DOI: 10.1007/s00534-004-0935-2

[55] Fatima J, Barton JG, Grotz TE, Geng Z, Harmsen WS, Huebner M, et al. Is there a role for endoscopic therapy as a definitive treatment for post-laparoscopic bile duct injuries? Journal of the American College of Surgeons. 2010; **211**(4):495-502. DOI: 10.1016/j.jamcollsurg.2010.06.013

[56] Zerem E, Omerović S. Minimally invasive management of biliary complications after laparoscopic cholecystectomy. European Journal of Internal Medicine. 2009;**20**(7):686-689. DOI: 10.1016/j.ejim.2009.07.010

[57] Walsh RM, Vogt DP, Ponsky JL, Brown N, Mascha E, Henderson JM. Management of failed biliary repairs for major bile duct injuries after laparoscopic cholecystectomy. Journal of the American College of Surgeons. 2004; **199**(2):192-197. DOI: 10.1016/j.jamcollsurg.2004.02.029

[58] Agarwal N, Sharma BC, Garg S, Kumar R, Sarin SK. Endoscopic management of postoperative bile leaks. Hepatobiliary & Pancreatic Diseases International. 2006;**5**(2):273-277

[59] ASGE Standards of Practice Committee, Chathadi KV, Chandrasekhara V, Acosta RD, Decker GA, Early DS, et al. The role of ERCP in benign diseases of the biliary tract. Gastrointestinal Endoscopy. 2015; **81**(4):795-803. DOI: 10.1016/j.gie.2014.11.019

[60] de Reuver PR, Rauws EA, Vermeulen M, Dijkgraaf MG, Gouma DJ, Bruno MJ. Endoscopic treatment of post-surgical bile duct injuries: Long term outcome and predictors of success. Gut. 2007;**56**(11):1599-1605. DOI: 10.1136/gut.2007.123596

[61] Gazzaniga GM, Filauro M, Mori L. Surgical treatment of iatrogenic lesions of the proximal common bile duct. World Journal of Surgery. 2001;**25**(10): 1254-1259. DOI: 10.1007/s00268-001-0105-5

[62] Pekolj J, Alvarez FA, Palavecino M, Sánchez Clariá R, Mazza O, de Santibañes E. Intraoperative management and repair of bile duct injuries sustained during 10,123 laparoscopic cholecystectomies in a high-volume referral center. Journal of the American College of Surgeons. 2013; **216**(5):894-901. DOI: 10.1016/j.jamcollsurg.2013.01.051

[63] Canena J, Horta D, Coimbra J, Meireles L, Russo P, Marques I, et al. Outcomes of endoscopic management of

primary and refractory postcholecystectomy biliary leaks in a multicentre review of 178 patients. BMC Gastroenterology. 2015;**15**:105. DOI: 10.1186/s12876-015-0334-y

[64] Pioche M, Ponchon T. Management of bile duct leaks. Journal of Visceral Surgery. 2013;**150**(3 Suppl):S33-S38. DOI: 10.1016/j.jviscsurg.2013.05.004

[65] Costamagna G, Pandolfi M, Mutignani M, Spada C, Perri V. Long-term results of endoscopic management of postoperative bile duct strictures with increasing numbers of stents. Gastrointestinal Endoscopy. 2001; **54**(2):162-168. DOI: 10.1067/mge.2001.116876

[66] Costamagna G, Tringali A, Perri V, Familiari P, Boškoski I, Barbaro F, et al. Endotherapy of postcholecystectomy biliary strictures with multiple plastic stents: Long-term results in a large cohort of patients. Gastrointestinal Endoscopy. 2020;**91**(1):81-89. DOI: 10.1016/j.gie.2019.05.042

[67] Schreuder AM, Busch OR, Besselink MG, Ignatavicius P, Gulbinas A, Barauskas G, et al. Long-term impact of iatrogenic bile duct injury. Digestive Surgery. 2020;**37**(1): 10-21. DOI: 10.1159/000496432

[68] Eum YO, Park JK, Chun J, Lee SH, Ryu JK, Kim YT, et al. Non-surgical treatment of post-surgical bile duct injury: Clinical implications and outcomes. World Journal of Gastroenterology. 2014;**20**(22): 6924-6931. DOI: 10.3748/wjg.v20.i22.6924

[69] de Jong EA, Moelker A, Leertouwer T, Spronk S, Van Dijk M, van Eijck CH. Percutaneous transhepatic biliary drainage in patients with postsurgical bile leakage and nondilated intrahepatic bile ducts. Digestive Surgery. 2013;**30**(4–6):444-450. DOI: 10.1159/000356711

[70] Jabłońska B, Lampe P, Olakowski M, Górka Z, Lekstan A, Gruszka T. Hepaticojejunostomy vs. end-to-end biliary reconstructions in the treatment of iatrogenic bile duct injuries. Journal of Gastrointestinal Surgery. 2009;**13**(6): 1084-1093. DOI: 10.1007/s11605-009-0841-7

[71] Thomson BN, Parks RW, Madhavan KK, Wigmore SJ, Garden OJ. Early specialist repair of biliary injury. The British Journal of Surgery. 2006; **93**(2):216-220. DOI: 10.1002/bjs.5194

[72] Huang Q, Yao HH, Shao F, Wang C, Hu YG, Hu S, et al. Analysis of risk factors for postoperative complication of repair of bile duct injury after laparoscopic cholecystectomy. Digestive Diseases and Sciences. 2014;**59**(12): 3085-3091. DOI: 10.1007/s10620-014-3255-7

[73] Maddah G, Rajabi Mashhadi MT, Parvizi Mashhadi M, Nooghabi MJ, Hassanpour M, Abdollahi A. Iatrogenic injuries of the extrahepatic biliary system. The Journal of Surgical Research. 2017;**213**:215-221. DOI: 10.1016/j.jss.2015.11.032

[74] Ismael HN, Cox S, Cooper A, Narula N, Aloia T. The morbidity and mortality of hepaticojejunostomies for complex bile duct injuries: A multi-institutional analysis of risk factors and outcomes using NSQIP. HPB: The Official Journal of the International Hepato Pancreato Biliary Association. 2017;**19**(4):352-358. DOI: 10.1016/j.hpb.2016.12.004

[75] Strasberg SM, Helton WS. An analytical review of vasculobiliary injury

in laparoscopic and open cholecystectomy. HPB (Oxford). 2011; **13**(1):1-14. DOI: 10.1111/j.1477-2574. 2010.00225.x

[76] de Santibañes E, Palavecino M, Ardiles V, Pekolj J. Bile duct injuries: Management of late complications. Surgical Endoscopy. 2006;**20**(11): 1648-1653. DOI: 10.1007/s00464-006-0491-8

[77] Strasberg SM, Gouma DJ. 'Extreme' vasculobiliary injuries: Association with fundus-down cholecystectomy in severely inflamed gallbladders. HPB (Oxford). 2012;**14**(1):1-8. DOI: 10.1111/j.1477-2574.2011.00393.x

[78] Truant S, Boleslawski E, Lebuffe G, Sergent G, Pruvot FR. Hepatic resection for post-cholecystectomy bile duct injuries: A literature review. HPB: The Official Journal of the International Hepato Pancreato Biliary Association. 2010;**12**(5):334-341. DOI: 10.1111/j.1477-2574.2010.00172.x